W9-CDS-368

SUDDEN DEATH
OF
ATHLETES

SUDDEN DEATH
OF
ATHLETES

By

ERNST JOKL, M.D., F.A.C.C.

University of Kentucky
College of Medicine
Lexington, Kentucky

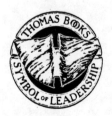

CHARLES C THOMAS • PUBLISHER
Springfield • Illinois • U.S.A.

Published and Distributed Throughout the World by

CHARLES C THOMAS • PUBLISHER
2600 South First Street
Springfield, Illinois 62717

With THOMAS BOOKS *careful attention is given to all details of manufacturing and design. It is the Publisher's desire to present books that are satisfactory as to their physical qualities and artistic possibilities and appropriate for their particular use.* THOMAS BOOKS *will be true to those laws of quality that assure a good name and good will.*

Printed in the United States of America
Q-R-3

Supported by
National Institutes of Health Grant LM 00009
from the National Library of Medicine
Bethesda, Maryland

Published on behalf of International Council of Sports
Sciences and Physical Education (UNESCO).

Library of Congress Cataloging in Publication Data

Jokl, Ernst, 1907-
    Sudden death of athletes.

    "Supported by the National Institutes of Health Grant LM00009
from the National Library of Medicine, Bethesda, Maryland" —
T.p. verso.
    Bibliography: p.
    Includes index.
    1. Heart — Diseases.   2. Athletes — Diseases.   3. Sudden
death.   I. National Library of Medicine (U.S.)   II. Title.
[DNLM: 1. Death, Sudden.   2. Exertion.   3. Sports Medicine.
QT 260 J75sa]
RC682.J65   1985   616.1'2   84-16295
ISBN 0-398-05088-0

To Marion and Peter

PREFACE

THE first study of cardiological aspects of athletics was conducted during the 1928 Olympic Games in Amsterdam. It was designed by Sir Adolphe Abrahams of London, Professor Isidor Snapper of Amsterdam, and Professor F.J.J. Buytendijk of Utrecht. S. Hoogerwerf, coworker of Willem Einthoven recorded electrocardiograms. F. Deutsch and H. Herxheimer took cardiac measurements from roentgenograms, and M. Burger applied cardiorespiratory stress tests. The results of the studies were published in 1929.[1]

During the early fifties long term research programs on sports cardiology were initiated by H. Reindell[2] of Freiburg, Germany and by Sir Adolphe Abrahams[3-5] of London. An epidemiological survey that included comparative analyses of coronary risk factors was conducted at the 1952 Olympic Games in Helsinki, Finland.[6] Two major studies of the problem of sudden death associated with exercise were undertaken by Moritz and Zamcheck[7] of the U.S. Army Institute of Pathology in Washington, D.C. and by Jokl and McClellan.[8]

The aim of this volume is to bring up-to-date earlier writings on the problem of fatal cardiac collapses associated with exercise. Their analysis necessitated consideration of a variety of clinical aspects of sports medicine elaborated in the book "Heart and Sport,"[233] in the above mentioned volume "Exercise and Cardiac Death" (with J.T. McClellan),[8] and in the monographs, "Heart and Sport"[233] and "Olympic Medicine and Sports Cardiology."[234] A discussion of sequelae of cardiac trauma in sport is contained in the book, "Medical Aspects of Boxing"[235]; elaborate descriptions of collapse syndromes of athletes in the monographs, "Zusammenbruche beim Sport"[155] and "Syncope in Athletes."[13] The Immunological Status of Athletes has been analyzed in a series of serological, clinical and epidemiological publications.[171,172,174] The question whether exercise is able to eliminate pathological processes has been dealt with in the introduction to "The Role of Exercise in Internal Medicine"[236] and in my Address to the Meeting of the New York Academy of Medicine in Commemoration of the Hundredth Anniversary of the Birth of Paul Ehrlich.[237]

Introduction

THE CONTRIBUTION OF CLINICAL
SPORTS MEDICINE TO CARDIOLOGY

CLINICAL studies with athletes have yielded information on six issues of relevance to cardiology.

First, concise evidence has been made available on structure and function of "athlete's heart" delineating it against the cardiomyopathies for which it is sometimes mistaken. The functional excellence of "athlete's heart" stands in contrast to the pathological nature of its counterpart.

Second, research in clinical sports medicine has clarified the problem of unexpected cardiac seizures and of sudden death associated with physical exertion. It has shown that fatalities during exercise are not caused by exercise. A fatal collapse during exercise may represent the first manifestation of cardiac disease identified only at autopsy. The discovery post mortem of disease processes in the heart does not always explain the pathophysiology of the events preceding the fatalities. Triggers responsible for the elicitation of the syncopal events have been described, chief among them intercurrent infections, trauma to the chest, and thermic stress. Cardiac seizures associated with exercise do not occur fortuitously. The extent to which they may be genetically programmed is indicated by the simultaneous occurrence of myocardial infarction in identical twins, or by unexpected deaths in members of several generations of the same family. The implications of the issue transcend their importance to sports medicine. They are of axiomatic significance to aviation medicine.

Third, clinical sports medicine has thrown light upon limitations of adaptability of the autonomic nervous system: observations of collapse syndromes after exhausting athletic effort have yielded insight into scope and limitation of vegetative regulation mechanisms: of acute attacks of migraine, cataplectic loss of muscle tone, orthostatic collapse, syncopal amnestic states and of failure of the body's temperature control mechanism. With the exception of the latter, these collapses do not cause fatalities in competitive athletes. But they reveal "break-points" of the body's homeostatic capacity. Sir William Osler's statement that "patients do not die of their disease: they die of physiologic abnormalities of their disease" receives corroboration in a new context.

Fourth, clinical research with athletes has shown that physical training fails to enhance immunological resistence. Actually, athletes are more susceptible than non-athletes to communicable diseases, viral, bacterial and parasitic. The widely held view that physical training engenders enhanced immunological powers is erroneous. The issue is of fundamental importance to sports medicine since the elimination of infectious diseases through medical measures has been one of the main causes of the athletic performance explosion that characterizes the contemporary sports movement.

Fifth, the problem of "the aging heart" had to be reviewed when massive evidence became available showing that advancing age is no obstacle to the attainment of good, at times even of superb athletic performances. A study of the physical and health status of 1,704 participants in the National Festival for Senior Gymnasts in Marburg, Germany undertaken in 1952 (age range of male participants — 40 to 82; women — 32 to 56) revealed that trained old people are fitter than untrained young subjects. Trained women maintain their physical performance potential unchanged between ages 30 and 45. At the Olympic Games in 1960, 1964, 1968, and 1972 a number of grandmothers, all of them strikingly young in appearance, obtained medals. In 1982, 47 women aged 55 and older finished the Honolulu marathon. Evidently, effective responses to training occur not only in healthy subjects but also in subjects afflicted with chronic cardiovascular and other illnesses, irrespective of age.

Sixth, the problem of the health value of exercise has been elucidated through clinical studies with athletes. Does exercise promote health? Is exercise able to eliminate pathological processes?

More than 100 years ago Julius Cohnheim,[18] the pathologist, contrasted adaptations in physiology and pathology. The latter, he pointed out, cannot be relied upon to fight disease processes. Contrariwise, physiological adaptations "serve their purpose": power training strengthens the musculature; endurance training enhances the capacity to perform over longer time; and training of skill improves the coordinative capacity of the motor system.

Cohnheim's ideas represent the conceptual basis for an understanding of the effectiveness of the use of exercise in cardiac rehabilitation: physiological adaptations to exercise take place in healthy as well as in chronically diseased subjects, including patients after myocardial infarction — provided they are able to exercise. Not all of them are. That physical power and mental well being are greatly improved through training is beyond doubt. However, a direct effect of exercise upon pathological processes in human subjects has not yet been observed. Exercise cannot remove plaques in the coronary arteries, nor scars in the myocardium.

Epidemiological evidence revealing a superior clinical and performance status of physically active subjects may well be explained by self selection plus the known effectiveness of training. Since severely ill patients abstain from exercise, a gradient of pathological involvement of the cardiovascular system may be reflected in corresponding levels of clinical status and of performance capacity ranging from dependence upon intensive care to participation in long distance running.

ACKNOWLEDGEMENTS

M Y thanks are due to the following authors from whose writings I have quoted: Thomas James (on cardioneuropathies), J.R. Green, L.J. Krovetz, D.R. Shanklin (on genetic defects of conduction system), D.L. Glancy and P. Yarnell (on traumatic aneurysm), R.W. Schrier, H.S. Henderson, C.C. Tisher, R.L. Tanner (on nephropathy and heat stress), L.G.C.E. Pugh (on hypothermia), F.L. Giknis, D.E. Holt, H.W. Whitemen, M.D. Sing, A. Benchimol. E.G. Dimond (on myocardial infarction in twins); A.A.J. Adgey (on cardiomyopathy). L. Melzer (on non-traumatic collapse), M.M. Suzman (on valvular disease in athletes), J. Greenstein (on fatal coronary sclerosis in a child), B. Newman (on death of a wrestler), E.H. Cluver (on death of a champion athlete), R.H. Mackintosh (on rupture of aorta); to G.E. Friend (on heart strain), A.R. Moritz and N. Zamcheck (on sudden death of young soldiers), I. Gore and O. Sphir (on myocarditis), A.L. Muir, I.W. Percy-Robb, J.A. Davidson, E.G. Walsh, R. Passmore (on observations during Edinburgh Commonwealth Games), E. Sohar, D. Michaeli, U. Waks, S. Shibolet, M.C. Lancaster, Y. Danon and C. Wyndham (on heat stroke), D.J. Dalessio (on effort migraine), Elizabeth Schickele (on heat stroke), E.C. Parker Williams (on poliomyelitis), Cerva, Novak and Culbertson (on amebic meningoencephalitis, D.F. Hanley (on observations with U.S. Olympic Team, and Ralph Paffenbarger and Daniel Brunner (on cardiological epidemiology).

CONTENTS

SUDDEN DEATH
OF
ATHLETES

Chapter I

ATHLETE'S HEART

Historical Review

PRIOR to the second half of the 19th century, it was generally believed that exercise was a potential cause of cardiac damage. In 1869, Prof. J.E. Morgan studied the after-health of 294 men who had rowed in the Oxford and Cambridge University Boat Race between the years of 1829 and 1869. Seventeen of them, he wrote, complained of "ill effects" whose nature, however, was not detailed. In a lecture at Edinburgh in 1883 entitled, "The Use and Abuse of Physical Training," C.W. Cathcart dealt with "the dangers to the heart of organized games in schools." In 1892, Sir Frederick Treves devoted twelve out of twenty pages of an article on medical aspects of exercise to a discussion of "heart strain from exercise," a problem which according to a statement made in 1893 by W. Collier had to be kept in mind in designing physical education programs for children. Sir Lauder Brunton, in an address to the York Medical Society in 1898 on medical aspects of athletics, emphasized "the vulnerability of the heart of young boys." In 1901 a London daily paper published a letter "signed by four eminent doctors" condemning all runs of over one mile by high school boys. Prior to 1900 girls were not mentioned. At the time the view was paramount that a "horse sweats, a man perspires, but a lady only glows." Though never substantiated, admonitions of the above mentioned kind impresssed the man on the street. To some extent they still do so today. An editorial in *The Lancet* of 28th May 1938, recalled that in 1909 five members of the

3

medical profession in England, including Sir Thomas Barlow and Sir William Hale-White started a correspondence in *The Times* by saying that "school and cross-country races exceeding one mile in distance are wholly unsuitable for boys under the age of 19, as the continued strain involved is apt to cause permanent injury to the heart and other organs." In the discussion that followed among medical officers of schools, the majority agreed with Sir Clifford Allbutt, who declared he had never had reason to suppose that any particular harm had been caused by exercise.[15]

In 1935, F.W. Lempriere analyzed medical records of 16,000 school boys covering a period of thirty years. This impressive study led to the conclusion which startled the medical profession that "heart strain through exercise is practically unknown." Lempriere mentioned six fatalities in twenty years, four of them due to accidents. Of the remaining two, one concerned a football player who died two hours after a meal; the other a boy who high jumped eight days after an attack of tonsillitis. His death took place "seven months later from infective endocarditis." No autopsies were made and the relation to exercise seemed remote. Mention was also made of a young girl who suffered a fatal collapse on the hockey field, presumably caused by heart failure following exercise after a heavy meal.

Friend[19] reviewed the entire medical information on heart and sport available in England until 1935. He pointed out that there is no evidence to support the view that exercise can cause cardiac damage. His report mentions that during the years following the foundation of the Medical Officers of Schools Association in England in 1884, more than 50 papers were published in *School Hygiene* from 1910 to 1912, in the *Journal of School Hygiene and Physical Education* from 1923 to 1926 and in the *Annual Reports of the Association* from 1926 to 1934, most containing warnings of "heart strain through exercise." In light of the facts as we know them, the papers read like Hans Christian Andersen's fairy tale of "The Emperor's Invisible Clothes." No clinical information nor autopsy protocols were presented during the long period under discussion to support the allegation that heart disease can be caused by exercise. In fact the hearts of young athletes are singularly capable to adapt themselves to strenuous exercise. This statement applies to children in general and to girls in particular; it is of exceptional relevance for the evaluation of athletic feats such as that of young adolescent girls who today dominate the Olympic competitions in gymnastics, swimming and ice skating, not to speak of children who participate in long distance runs. Many current athletic records have been established by adolescent boys and girls. There can be no doubt that the medical prophets of doom quoted in the foregoing possessed more eloquence than knowledge.

The resources of scientific medicine were only recently brought to bear upon the study of the problem of heart and sport. Specifically it was the clarification of six issues that made a mark upon clinical cardiology: the elucidation of the differential diagnostic characteristics of the pathologically enlarged heart as against the physiologically adapted heart of the endurance athlete; the description of exhaustion syndromes after maximal athletic performances; the analysis of cardiac seizures and of fatal collapses associated with exercise; the elucidation of the role of exercise in gerontology; the understanding of scope and limitation of the therapeutic use of exercise in clinical cardiology and in cardiac rehabilitation; and of the immunological status of athletes.

"Cor bovinum"

In 1849 Prof. Carl von Rokitansky[14] of Vienna referred to the large heart of patients with arterial hypertension as "ox-heart" or "cor bovinum." At autopsy he found grossly hypertrophied hearts, some of them weighing more than 1,000 g. Such enormous hypertrophy of the ventricles leads to a critical reduction of the blood supply of the myocardium whose failure causes the patients' premature death. It is against the background of these pathological studies that the concern over "athlete's heart" expressed by the early representatives of sports medicine around the turn of our century must be interpreted. Many of them thought that intensive physical training gives rise to the development of the "cor bovinum" as described by Rokitansky. In support of their theories they quoted semi-mythological accounts of fatal collapses due to physical exertion, often including that of the "Runner of Marathon," who reportedly died on the market square of Athens in the year 490 B.C. after bringing the news of the defeat of the Persian invaders by the heroic Greek armies under the command of Miltiades. The story appealed and continues to appeal to the imagination of the man on the street. In 1957, one of the most respected American medical journals published an article on marathon running from which the following is taken:

> I wonder if death is not a vague ultimate aim of marathoners. They run to the point of utter exhaustion; marathon runners are essentially messengers, at least most of the ancient ones were, and they were always so seriously intent on the King's business that they ran themselves into collapse. It is traditional for all worthy messengers to take a fierce pride in their endurance and to run to a point of collapse and death. This motif occurs again and again in literature. In the *Incident of the French Camp*, by Robert Browning, the young messenger came whipping into camp to bring word to Napoleon of the progress of some distant battle. But no sooner had he completed his task when he perished:
>
> > *"You're wounded!" Nay, the soldier's pride*
> > *Touched to the quick, he said;*
> > *"I'm kill'd, Sire!" And his chief beside,*
> > *Smiling the boy fell dead.*
>
> One always sees in these messengers a moment of exaltation when they have finally won through and delivered the news, and then it seems to be an almost inexorable destiny for them to drop dead — anything but death would be dull, sudden anticlimax.

A fanciful assertion presented in the disguise of profound learnedness.

Henschen's Report in 1899

The first description of the "heart of the athlete" *(Sportherz)* as a functionally superior organ characterized by large size as well as excellent performance capacity was published in German. It appeared in Volume II of *Mitteilungen aus der Medizinischen Klinik zu Upsala* (Sweden) in 1899 and was written by S.E. Henschen,[20] Professor of Medicine at the University of Upsala. The title of the report was: *"Eine medizinische Sportstudie; Skidlauf und Skidwettlauf."* ("A Study in Sports Medicine; Skiing and Competitive Skiing") Using manual percussion of the chest wall — roentgenology was at the time in its infancy — Henschen noticed that the majority of successful contestants in long distance skiing races had exceptionally large hearts. The largest hearts he encountered were in the winners of the *"Gefle-Forsbacka"* and the *"Falu"* — races over distances of 25 and 95 k respectively.

In interpreting his findings, Henschen introduced the now generally understood distinction between the functionally efficient large heart of successful endurance athletes, as against the pathologically enlarged heart of patients with cardiomyopathy in whom it is indicative of progressive disease.

The 1928 Olympic Medical Study

A scientific assessment of the status of heart of athletes was made during the 1928 Olympic Games in Amsterdam, by F.J.J. Buytendijk of Utrecht, and Herbert Herxheimer of Berlin.[1] Chest x-ray pictures revealed significantly enlarged hearts in competitors in endurance events, e.g., running, cycling and swimming. Since then, H. Reindell[2] of Freiburg has examined the hearts of hundreds of athletes and non-athletes. He confirmed the validity of the results of the 1928 Olympic study and supplied additional information: physical endurance and cardiac size are correlated.

Roentgenological and echocardiographic assessment of cardiac size must be carried out with the subject lying since orthostatic displacement of blood renders measurement with the subject standing unreliable. The magnitude of cardiac enlargement accompanying intensive endurance training can be considerable. Relative to body weight the heart of endurance athletes can double in size. The largest athlete's heart known is that of the world record long distance runner, Henry Rono (capacity 200.8 ml/kg body weight).

The existence of a physiologic limit of adaptive enlargement of the heart in athletes active in endurance sports is shown by the fact that notwithstanding the great increase of volume of training during the past decades, the hearts of today's athletes are not larger than those measured three decades ago by Reindell.

Adaptive Responses

Under the influence of training, the capacity of the cardiovascular system to transport oxygen improves, first due to an increase of mitochondrial mass in skeletal muscles, accompanied by a decrease of catecholamine levels in blood and tissues and increase of left ventricular stroke volume. Contrariwise, diminution of left ventricular stroke volume due to pathological enlargement of the cardiomyopathic heart is accompanied by a rise of catecholamine levels.[21,22,23]

The adaptive changes which the hearts of athletes undergo during training represent but one of many facets of a physiological adjustment of the autonomic nervous system in its entirety. The organism of trained endurance athletes is distinguished by a preponderance of parasympathetic tone, to which Paul Dudley White first drew attention.[9] Sinus-bradycardia, now a well recognized normal phenomenon in athletes, is usually accompanied by A-V nodal bradycardia of proportionate degree. As the A-V nodal pacemaker has a slower automaticity than the sinus pacemaker it is usually not manifest electrocardiographically. Schamroth and Jokl[24] have studied electrocardiograms of a champion long distance runner with a resting bradycardia of under 40 in whom concommitant A-V nodal and sinus bradycardia with greater depression of sinus automaticity led to a dominant A-V nodal rhythm with *interference-dissociation.* Cardiac enlargement and bradycardia in athletes reflect increased parasympathetic tone, a physiologically appropriate adjustment. Both are reversible. Its corresponding opposite is the increased sympathetic tone accompanied by elevated levels of catecholamines in subjects with reduced exercise capacity. The prognostic significance of the latter category in respect to ischemic heart diseases was shown by W. Raab.[25]

To reiterate: contestants in *endurance* sports have distinctly enlarged hearts, while hearts of contestants in *power* sports are of normal size. The adaptive nature of the enlargement of the heart of endurance athletes is shown by the fact that myocardial mass decreases relative to body size; myocardial mass of hearts of athletes excelling in power sports increases though invariably within physiological limits.[2] Morganroth, et al.[26,27] have presented results of echocardiographic studies of hearts of trained distance runners and wrestlers. The latters' hearts were found to be of normal size, with their left ventricular walls and interventricular septa thickened; while, as expected, the end-diastolic volumes of hearts of distance runners were larger than those of sedentary subjects. Discontinuation of training causes the hearts of athletes to revert to normal. No such reversal of size and mass occurs in hearts with pathologically hypertrophied myocardium.

Physiological Enlargement of Myocardium

According to Maron, et al.[28,29] the diagnosis of hypertrophic cardiomyopathy presupposes presence of at least one of the following features: asymmetric septal hypertrophy; marked disorganization of cardiac muscle cells in the ventricular septum; and evidence of hypertrophic cardiomyopathy in family members. None of these is associated with athlete's heart. The latter never causes death, the former does. Pathological hypertrophy of myocardium may develop secondary to myocarditis, to coronary disease, to congenital anomalies of heart and blood vessels, also to aortic and subaortic stenosis. Hypertrophic cardiomyopathy is never caused by athletic training.[30]

Cardiomyopathic hearts and large hearts of endurance athletes differ greatly: the former reflect a critical impairment of its functional capacity, the latter optimal adaptation; the former may weigh as much as 1,000 g, the latter rarely more than 500 g; the former impede exercise capacity, the latter facilitate it; the former grow progressively in size, the latter establish a steady-state level once they reach their appropriate form; the former herald early death, the latter signify superior cardiac health. For the small heart of the physically inactive city dweller, Wilhelm Raab[25] has coined the term, "loafer's heart."

Girl Swimmers' Hearts

In order to excel in endurance events, it is of great advantage to an athlete to be genetically endowed with a large heart whose size is further increased through training. Swedish girl swimming champions examined by Astrand, et al.[31] had hearts considerably larger than those of an untrained control group. Four years after discontinuation of their competitive careers, the girls' hearts were still conspicuously large though their maximal oxygen intake capacity had diminished. Presumably, they had been large at the time they took up their sport. Under the influence of training their powers of endurance became correspondingly superior as a result of cardiac as well as extracardiac adaptation.

Reversibility of Adaptive Cardiac Enlargement

Roentgenograms taken in 1925 from one of the world's best known long distance cyclists, Walter Ruett at the height of his racing career and again twelve years after his retirement, revealed that cessation of training had caused a distinct reduction of the size of his heart. In a monograph entitled, "Response to Exercise after Bed Rest," B. Saltin, et al.[32] described observations on healthy young athletes who participated in an experiment in which circulatory responses to exercise were recorded before and after twenty-one days of bed rest. A significant reduction of the size of the heart occurred in every subject during their inactivity. It took sixty days of training to reestablish their initial cardiac status.

Exercise and Life Expectancy

Several attempts have been made to answer the question whether exercise prolongs life. Pyorala, Karvonen, Taskinen, Takkunen and Kyronseppa[33,34] investigated the cardiac status of sixty-one former champion long-distance skiers of ages 40-79. Their results suggested that the endurance training of the skiers had prolonged their lives by five to seven years. In discussing their findings, the Finnish authors wrote:

> In their later years, former endurance athletes are susceptible to cardiovascular diseases just as aging people are who had not engaged in sports. But the incidence of heart disease in the ex-athletes was distinctly smaller than in the latter group.

Another study directed by Karvonen, et al.[35] aimed at an assessment of longevity of a group of skiers compiled from the best participants in the Oulu race during the years 1889-1930. The mortality of the skiers was followed until 1967 and compared to that of the general male population. Statistical evaluation of the data revealed a difference in longevity of 2.8 years in favor of the skiers.

The sixty-one former champion long distance skiers as well as the former participants in the Oulu race represented epidemiologically selected samples in that their cardiovascular status can be assumed to have been superior to that of the general population of the age range under study, in terms of physiological as well as pathological criteria. A true prolongation of the life span is not engenered by physical activity although it is true that athletes adhere to a life style in which the chief coronary risk factors do not play the same role as they do in non-athletes.

One of the most comprehensive studies of longevity of former athletes was undertaken by Rook[36] who evaluated information obtained on former Cambridge students who had represented their University in contests with Oxford at rowing, cricket, rugby, and track-and-field athletics from 1860 to 1900. He compared the data with data of non-athletic Cambridge students. The length of life of the athletes did not differ from that of the controls.

Chapter II

SUDDEN AND UNEXPECTED DEATH

If a person died during exercise he did not die from exercise. (E. Jokl and J. T. McClellan)

Moritz and Zamcheck's Study

In 1946 Moritz and Zamcheck[7] presented the results of a study on "Sudden and Unexpected Death of Young Soldiers" based upon an analysis of autopsy results received by the Army Institute of Pathology between 1942 and 1946 of apparently healthy soldiers who had unexpectedly died from heart disease. The study dealt with post mortem findings in 145 cases of fatal collapses: 115 from disease of the coronary arteries; 14 from myocarditis; six from syphilitic aortitis; five from rheumatic heart disease; and five from myocardial fibrosis.

Autopsy Findings

Coronary Artery Disease: In 98 of the 115 unexpected deaths from disease of the coronary arteries, the type of physical activity that had preceded or accompanied the onset of the fatal seizure was recorded: in 29% its onset coincided with strenuous physical exertion. Comparison of estimated time devoted by soldiers to inactivity and to activity to the number of fatal seizures coincident with inactivity or activity led to the conclusion that if a young man is to die unexpectedly of coronary disease, the onset of the fatal attack is more likely to take place during strenuous physical exertion than during sleep.

12

Coronary thrombosis was found in 31 cases, obliterative coronary sclerosis in 23, and severe coronary arteriosclerosis without thrombosis or obliteration in 61. Myocardial infarction was seen in 22 cases and myocardial fibrosis without infarction in 27. In 66 cases there was no myocardial pathology. Cardiac hypertrophy (defined by heart weight greater than 400 g) was encountered in 33 out of the 115 cases.

Myocarditis: In 14 instances, death had resulted from diffuse or focal exudative inflammation of the myocardium. Ten of the 14 died within a few minutes after an unexpected syncopal attack. In two, the fatal seizure occurred during a period of strenuous physical exertion; eight were at rest or engaged in ordinary activity.

Syphilitic Aortitis: In six cases of sudden death active syphilitic inflammation of the aortic ring was found post mortem. Of these, four died after unexpected syncopal attacks during ordinary activity.

Rheumatic Heart Disease. Five unexpected deaths were attributed to rheumatic heart disease. Four of them collapsed unexpectedly during periods of physical exertion.

Idiopathic Myocardial Fibrosis: Five deaths were attributed to acute cardiac failure due to extensive myocardial fibrosis not associated with coronary disease, myocarditis, or rheumatic heart disease. In three of the five cases, there was cardiac hypertrophy.

Mention is made of "aortic rupture" as possible cause of sudden death, no further detail being given.

Characteristics of Fatal Seizures in 96 Witnessed Cases

	Cases
Simple syncope*	68
Convulsions	17
Substernal or epigastic pain and syncope	9
Headache and syncope	2

In addition to the findings corresponding to those presented by Moritz and Zamcheck[7] the following pathological conditions have been seen by Jokl and McClellan[8] in *persons who had died in association with exercise:*

a) Congenital anomalies of coronary arteries;

---

* Rarely preceded by vomiting or followed by labored respiration.

b) Lesions of the Purkinje-His-system;
c) Hypoplasia of the arterial system;
d) Cardiac tumors;
e) Cardiac aftermath of athletic trauma.

Jokl and McClellan's Study [8,37]

The clarification of the problem of sudden cardiac death associated with physical exertion represents the most important single contribution made by clinical sportsmedicine to internal medicine so far. It is now possible to differentiate between the natural history of heart disease in patients who during their illness seek medical advice, as contrasted to that of persons in whom the terminal collapse represents the first manifestation of the cardiac affliction.

The ensuing case descriptions pertain to clinical observation and findings at autopsy of subjects who experienced cardiac seizures or died in association with exercise. They have been selected because they represent the diagnostic entities under discussion.

CORONARY ARTERY DISEASE

Even at the age of highest sport activities one is not protected against myocardial infarctions. (H. Roskamm, H. Gohlke, et al.[38])

The frequency with which the onset of fatal attacks of coronary insufficiency occurs during a period of strenuous physical exertion lends support to the prevalent and plausible opinion that violent exercise is probably dangerous for persons suffering from severe coronary disease. (A.R. Moritz, N. Zamcheck)

The most frequent cause of exertional angina and of sudden and unexpected death in association with exercise is coronary artery disease.

Death of a Wrestler

A 45-year-old wrestler complained of pressure in his chest immediately after a contest. He died in the dressing room a few minutes later. He had wrestled competitively for over 20 years; had never been seriously ill; and had not complained of symptoms referable to his heart.

Autopsy revealed a heart weighing 250 grams. The left coronary artery which showed severe atherosclerosis with ulceration was occluded by a semi-firm non-adherent thrombus. The right coronary artery was almost completely stenosed by calcified atheromatous plaques and cholesterol clefts. Microscopic examination revealed numerous focal areas of myocardial degeneration with patches of fibrous replacement. No inflammatory infiltrate was present.[39]

The case exemplifies the possibility of a mortal cardiac disease developing asymptomatically and without major reduction of physical performance capacity.

Death of a Child after Boxing

A 10-year-old boy collapsed and died five minutes after a boxing match lasting three rounds. He had received a number of blows against chest and abdomen but was not knocked down, nor did he seem to be unduly distressed at any time during the fight. At autopsy the left descending branch of the coronary artery was blocked for a distance of about one inch, beginning 1/2 inch from the orifice. Above and below the occlusion were atheromatous changes in the intima. Histological examination of the diseased portion of the coronary artery revealed an almost complete occlusion. The intima was thickened and hyalinised and an organized thrombus occupied the lumen of the vessel. There was marked cellular activity inside the thrombus. Several plaques of calcium were deposited between intima and media; the surrounding tissues were infiltrated with erythrocytes.[40]

The cause of the coronary artery disease responsible for the fatality could not be established. The case related to one of the youngest subjects known to have died from coronary heart disease in association with athletic exercise.

Death of a Pilot

A 50-year-old pilot of a passenger plane complained during the flight of shortness of breath. A few minutes later he slumped over dead. A passenger landed the plane. On the morning of the day of his death, he had played 18 holes of golf. At autopsy, an aneurysmatic bulge was noted near the apex. The left branch of the coronary artery was occluded in two places by thrombi: one red-brown and without signs of organization, the other organized. The circumflex artery was totally obstructed by atheromatous plaques. The right coronary artery was blocked over a distance of half an inch by a fresh massive hemorrhage into an organized atheromatous plaque. The myocardium of the left ventricle near the apex showed reddish discoloration suggestive of infarction. Scattered fibrous scars measuring up to one centimeter in diameter were noted in septum and wall of the left ventricle.[41]

The case illustrates the central importance of the problem of unexpected sudden cardiac death for aviation medicine. It also shows that seemingly unimpaired physical performance capacity need not necessarily signify cardiac integrity.

Death of Competitive Athletes

Tunstall-Pedoe[42] saw a fatal collapse due to previously undiagnosed coronary heart disease in a professional football player during a game. Waller and Roberts[43] described five cases of fatal collapse during running. The subjects whose ages were between 40 and 53 had participated in competitive running events. In all five cases autopsy revealed critical narrowing of the left anterior descending and of the circumflex coronary arteries. Four of the subjects had not experienced signs or symptoms of coronary artery disease; one who had suffered from angina before he died had completed six Boston marathons and several 80 kilometer runs.

In-flight Myocardial Infarction

In a report on sudden incapacitation in the United States Air Force, Rayman and MacNaughton[44] refer to five cases of suspected in-flight myocardial infarction. One occurred after touchdown with the navigator taking control of the aircraft; another during approach and landing, the co-pilot taking over. In a third case of suspected infarction the pilot had chest pain followed by loss of consciousness and death in flight. Infarctions were also suspected in a pilot who was killed in a crash, and in another instance in a navigator.

Myocardial Infarction in Identical Twins

Giknis, et al.[45] reported the occurrence of myocardial infarction in twenty-year-old identical twins: in the one during bowling and in the other after lifting a large pipe. Both had been athletically inclined, had put on boxing exhibitions in childhood. Their physical conditions were considered excellent. In twin I the clinical diagnosis of inferior myocardial infarction with lateral involvement was verified by laboratory and ECG evidence.

The second twin who lived distant from his brother had a sudden impulse to go home, sensing something was wrong. When he arrived and saw his brother hospitalized, he experienced constricting anterior chest pain, nausea, and dyspnea. He was admitted to the hospital where anterolateral myocardial infarction was diagnosed. Angiography revealed medium-sized narrowing of the left coronary artery. A year later the twins were re-examined. Both were found symptom-free and working regularly. (See also references 46 and 70.)

Coronary Artery Disease in Marathon Runner

Handler, et al.[47] described a case of symptomatic coronary artery disease in a 48-year-old marathon runner in whom coronary angiography revealed complete obstruction of the left anterior descending coronary artery and ventricular hypertrophy.

MYOCARDITIS

Death of a Long Distance Runner

After competing in a 12 mile cross-country race in which he placed 22nd among 62 runners, a 25-year-old soldier collapsed and died. He had been known to be a good athlete, having distinguished himself over several years in gymnastic competitions.

The deceased's personal files contained a report of a medical examination conducted a few days before his death, saying that no abnormalities were detected, and that a urine examination had yielded normal results. However, it was recorded that 10 weeks earlier he had contracted a gonorrhoeic urethritis which at the time of examination was believed to have been healed.

At autopsy, islands of connective tissue were scattered throughout the myocardium, histologically identified as due to sub-acute myocarditis. Interstitial infiltrates containing histiocytes and plasma cells were seen. Hyaline degeneration of the intima caused narrowing of the caliber of the small branches of the coronary arteries only. The main branches of the coronary arteries were unaffected.[48]

Gonorrhoeic myocarditis and endocarditis were not uncommon findings at autopsy during the pre-antibiotic era. In a monograph published in 1898, G. Kolb[49] discussed in a special chapter, *"Gonorrhoische Endokarditis bei Meistern im Wettrudern"* ("Gonorrhoeic endocarditis in Champion Oarsmen").

Myocarditis Simulating Myocardial Infarction

Acute infectious myocarditis or myopericarditis may simulate non-transmural myocardial infarction. A case in point in the report by Hanson, et al.[50] on a national class swimmer in the 200 meter butterfly event who complained of severe substernal chest pain while performing a 15 kilometer training session and who was believed to have suffered myocardial infarction. Myocardial infarction in a national class swimmer is an extremely unusual occurrence. No previous case of myocardial infarction in an Olympic class finalist in running or swimming has been observed. Other fatalities said by Hanson, et al. to have occurred "after vigorous physical activity"[51,52,53] did not follow physical performances of a magnitude comparable to that during which the episode reported by Hanson, et al. occurred.

In a comment on Hanson, et al.'s report, Karjalainen and Heikkila[54] wrote that the patient's episode of substernal pain must have been due to myocarditis. Hanson, et al.'s report contains no evidence of coronary atherosclerosis or spasm; serial ECGs showed changes typical of acute pericarditis as well as widespread initial ST-segment elevation, followed by localized T-wave inversion; no Q-waves were in evidence despite a conspicuous elevation of creatine kinase MB level. Creatine kinase MB elevation, Karjalainen and Heikkila write, is detected in 70% of patients who have acute myopericarditis with ST-segment elevation. The enzyme release simulates that in myocardial infarction but it is of short duration, not exceeding six days. Ventriculographic and echocardiographic evidence suggests that myocardial dysfunction in myocarditis is often local, and that uninvolved myocardial segments are hypercontractile, as in the present case.

Four weeks after his discharge the patient is reported to have regained his previous level of athletic performances — complete functional restitution is unlikely to take place with such rapidity after myocardial infarction.

RHEUMATIC HEART DISEASE

Acute Incapacitation of Racing Cyclist

A 21-year-old racing cyclist fell during a training ride, hurting his left knee. There was no open injury. On the following day the knee joint was swollen. A few days later all the other joints were swollen; temperature had risen to 104°F. The patient was admitted to the hospital where he was told that he suffered from rheumatic fever and that his heart was affected. Within the following three weeks the swelling of the joints subsided and temperature returned to normal; however, "the heart remained bad." The patient suffered from "stitch" in the cardiac region and dyspnea on slight exertion. In spite of his disability he tried to continue with his cycle racing but could no longer perform. His general condition deteriorated. He suffered from dyspnea, tachycardia, thirst and nocturia.

Before the accident he had won a number of major cycling competitions, was known for his strength in mountainous territory. On one occasion he had covered 240 meters in seven hours. A few weeks before the accident he had won a race leading over 170 kilometers. His athletic career came literally to a standstill when during a training ride he became sick, had to dismount and fainted. When he regained consciousness he suffered from headache, felt nauseous, was short of breath and had to rest for one hour before he could ride home. A diagnosis of mitral insufficiency of rheumatic origin was made. The exacerbation of the illness had been initiated by the injury to the knee joint.

The medical history yielded information to the effect that between ages 9 and 21 he had apparently been healthy, had excelled in his strenuous sport. At age 8 he had suffered from St. Vitus Dance. In all probability he had harbored a latent rheumatic infection which was mobilized by the joint injury. After the illness following his fall he tried to continue with his bicycle racing. It was the syncope to which reference has been made, rather than the preceding symptoms of the cardiac disease, the dyspnea, tachycardia, thirst, and nocturia that compelled him to seek medical advice. During the ensuing five years the condition failed to improve.[55]

"Cardiac" Marathon Runner

In 1940 Jokl and Suzman[56] presented a paper, "Aortic Regurgitation and Mitral Stenosis in a Marathon Runner," with special reference to the effect of valvular heart disease on physical efficiency. It dealt with the case of a 32-year-old competitor at the marathon race held at Johannesburg at an altitude of 6,000 feet above sea level who was noted to have both systolic and diastolic murmurs at the apex and base of the heart, and a diffuse and markedly forcible impulse. He had competed in many marathon races in the past without ill effects and saw no reason why he should not run. He came fourth out of a field of 17, in a time of two hours, 50 minutes.

At the age of 9 he had rheumatic fever, his "joints were swollen and painful." Soon afterwards he contracted pneumonia. In the following years he was constantly ill with intestinal trouble and bilharzia. For a long time he passed blood in the urine. At age 19 rheumatic fever recurred. In spite of being weak he played rugby and on one occasion collapsed during a game and was taken in an unconscious state to a hospital with a temperature of 104°F. He spent the ensuing four months in the hospital. His legs were now atrophied to such an extent that he had to walk with crutches. Shortly afterwards he contracted malaria which was "treated successfully with quinine and brandy." At the age of 25 he was involved in an automobile accident in which he received severe burns over the chest and his right knee joint was pierced by a fragment of metal. A short time later he underwent an operation for a hernia.

His athletic history included fourteen marathon races, among them a winning performance in the 1934 elimination race for the British Empire Games. On two occasions he entered the annual 54 mile race from Durban to Pietermaritzburg, his record time being eight hours, 20 minutes. On numerous occasions he had run from Johannesburg to Pretoria, a distance of 36 miles. He also played squash and ranked as one of the best players in Johannesburg.

Examination of the heart confirmed the diagnosis of aortic regurgitation and mitral stenosis. Roentgenological examination showed no enlargement of the heart, especially no left ventricular hypertrophy. EKG studies failed to reveal signs of myocardial ischemia.

On three occasions attacks of fainting were observed, one during a cross country race, the other two during routine training sessions.

Warfield's Review

In a review of the result of examination of some 40,000 young recruits at a military camp in 1918, Warfield[57] referred to "a number of youths with aortic insufficiency who were athletes, some record holders who were unaware that they had any heart lesion." Similar observations were reported in the German literature after World War I, among them several relating to athletes with mitral stenosis and aortic regurgitation of mitral origin in whom no signs of decompensation were present.

CARDIOMYOPATHY

Sudden death after sport has been widely documented, but there is no proof that the relation is more than fortuitous. (P. Lynch[58])

Death Due to Hypertrophic Cardiomyopathy

A 15-year-old boy collapsed while running along a pavement being pursued by other boys. A nurse who came to his assistance found him pulseless and apnoeic. External cardiac massage and mouth-to-mouth respiration were started. A mobile coronary care unit arrived nine minutes later. By this time the boy had ventricular fibrillation. Counter-shocks across the chest wall restored sinus rhythm and consciousness.

Fifteen months later, the boy ran for a bus and collapsed in the street. He was transported to a nearby hospital in an unconscious state. Ventricular fibrillation was present and corrected. Subsequently, he showed evidence of cerebral damage and of left ventricular failure. Death occurred within 24 hours. Post mortem examination revealed gross hypertrophy of the left ventricular myocardium. Heart weighed 1,105 g. The interventricular septum encroached upon the cavity of the right ventricle.[59]

Maron's Reports

In 1978 and 1980 Maron, et al.[28,29] published two papers, one

entitled "Sudden Death in Patients with Hypertrophic Cardiomyopathy: Characterization of 26 Patients without Functional Limitation"; the other "Sudden Death in Young Athletes." Both discussed
evidence culled from case records of the National Heart, Lung and
Blood Institute, Armed Forces Institute of Pathology Cardiovascular Registry, United Hospitals-Miller Division Cardiovascular Registry, and Children's Hospital of Pittsburgh, and from news media.
The "Circumstances of Death" described by the author of the 26 patients: "Hiking" (case 1), "stepped out of school bus" (case 2), "mild
calisthenics" (case 3), "light play" (case 4), "sedentary activity" (case
8), and "throwing a football" (case 20); do not justify the statement
that prior to their fatal collapses the subjects were "without functional limitation."

Maron's second paper mentions the following autopsy findings:
atherosclerotic coronary disease; ruptured aorta; anomalous origin
of left coronary artery; hypoplastic coronary arteries; and hypertrophic cardiomyopathy. Like findings have been reported before.[8] Maron, et al.'s[28] sample (26 cases) includes no cases of
myocarditis, of endocarditis, of congenital subaortic stenosis, of cardiac tumors and of cardiac sequelae of athletic trauma. "Our data,"
Maron, et al. write, "cannot be used to define prevalence of diseases
causing death in athletes."[29] It would be of interest to read the
athletic histories of the 14 subjects who are described as having died
from hypertrophic cardiomyopathy. Were endurance athletes among
them? I have never seen at autopsy, hearts with hypertrophic cardiomyopathy in athletes who had competed in running or swimming
or skiing over extended distances. Can a heart afflicted with hyper-
torphic cardiomyopathy comply with the demands of long lasting
athletic contests? The condition referred to in Maron, et al.'s paper
showing the heart of a "13-year-old football and baseball player" is
very similar to that presented by Jokl in 1980,[39] relating to the findings at autopsy of a boy whose physical performance capacity had
been severely limited. He could definitely not have been described
as an athlete.

"Athlete's Heart" Versus Cardiomyopathy

Doubt as to the validity of statements to the effect that physiological adaptation of the heart to training can result in cardiomyopathy

has already been expressed.[60] Cardiac hypertrophy secondary to lesions such as congenital anomalies of the coronary arteries or congenital sub-aortic stenosis is not synonymous with "idiopathic hypertrophic cardiomyopathy," a distinction that will have to be maintained. The German school of sports cardiologists led by Linzbach[30] and Reindell[2] maintains that 500 g represent the "critical weight of the heart" in that hearts that weigh more than 500 g are not likely to be able to sustain top level athletic performances.

The question arises whether it is justified to say that the heart of a healthy long distance runner can be indistinguishable from a heart with hypertrophic cardiomyopathy. There are decisive differences between the two in respect of left ventricular wall performance, ejection fraction and volume. And last, but not least: hypertrophic cardiomyopathy is a cause of unexpected death; athlete's heart is not.

CONGENITAL ANOMALIES OF THE ARTERIAL SYSTEM

Supravalvular Aortic Stenosis, Aortic Rupture

A well-built athlete, aged 15, returned from a gymnastic class during which he had indulged in weight-lifting and wrestling. On reaching home he collapsed with a vice-like pain in the chest and died within an hour.

Autopsy showed the pericardium to be tense and bluish. It contained 150 ml of coagulated blood and 650 ml of fluid blood and hemorrhagic serum. The left ventricle was dilated and hypertrophied, being twice the normal size. The foramen ovale was closed, all three cusps of the aortic valves were present. The ductus arteriosus was patent and filled with a fresh thrombus. The isthmus of the aorta was so narrow that it admitted only a fine metal sound. Above the stenotic part the aorta was considerably dilated, forming a flaccid aneurysmal bag which bulged towards the right side. There was a tear three centimeters long in the lateral wall of this bag, starting just above the aortic valves and establishing a communication between the lumen of the aorta and the pericardium. The internal mammary arteries were much enlarged, their caliber corresponding to that of normal adult males. Below the stenosis the aorta was about half the normal width. Its walls were abnormally thin. No arteriosclerosis or atheroma was noted. No fibrous patches were seen in the myocardium.

A persistent thymus gland, weighing 38.4 grams, with active Hassall's corpuscles was found. There was an abundance of lymphatic tissue, especially in the spleen and the mesentery. Large lymphatic plaques were noted in the mucosa of the small intestine.[61]

This case is characterized by the presence of multiple congenital anomalies of which the stenosis of the isthmus of the aorta is the most important. This stenosis formed a mechanical obstruction, which explains the dilation of the aorta above the isthmus, the compensatory over-development of the internal mammary arteries, and the hypertrophy of the left ventricle. A persistent thymus gland with active Hassall's corpuscles, hypoplastic thin-walled arteries, and a general abundance of lymphatic tissue were found. The immediate cause of death was rupture of the ascending aorta.

The deceased had been a first-class athlete. Bonnet[62] has pointed out that, in the presence of isthmus stenosis, collateral circulation may compensate for the central defect. Hart[63] has reported on the sudden death of a man, aged 41, who prior to the fatal collapse was engaged in strenuous physical labor. Necropsy revealed complete obliteration of the isthmus, thromboendocarditis of a two-cusped aortic valve, mesaortitis syphilitica of the thoracic portion of the aorta, and hypertrophy of the left ventricle. Above the obliterated isthmus the aorta showed a "balloon-like" enlargement.

Wasastjerna[64] reported on a case of aortic rupture of a boy, aged 13, who had collapsed while skating. Jores[65] emphasized the general significance of physical effort in cases of rupture of the aorta in persons with stenosis of the aortic isthmus and ventricular hypertrophy. He said that, provided a good collateral circulation was established, exercise would not cause a rupture unless there was aneurysmal enlargement of the aorta and abnormal thinness of the artery walls. Arteriosclerosis is usually not present in cases of this kind, even though the elastic elements of the artery walls are as a rule affected.

The condition is rare; among 5,000 necropsies conducted between 1900 and 1905 by the Vienna Medico-Legal Institute, only four instances of advanced stenosis of the aortic isthmus were encountered. (A good general discussion of the issue can be found in the volume edited by Henke and Lubarsch.[66])

The question arises as to what part the weight-lifting and wrestling played in causing the fatal tear of the aorta in the present instance. The increase of arterial pressure accompanying activities of the kind under reference may well have caused the final rupture.

Aortic Stenosis

A 28-year-old man collapsed and died during a table tennis game. He had previously been believed to be healthy. At autopsy his heart weighed 620 g. Ventricular walls and intraventricular septum were markedly hypertrophied. The aortic valve was composed of three leaflets, all of them densely calcified, rigid and stenotic. The opening of the aortic valve measured eight millimeters in diameter; there was fresh thrombus formation on the valve surfaces. The other cardiac valves were normal. Microscopic examination of the myocardium revealed no fibrosis; the coronary arteries showed no atherosclerotic changes.

Aortic stenosis is usually the result of acquired disease. However, if the abnormal calcification is confined to the aortic valves the condition is almost sure to be a congenital malformation. Taussig[67] writes that congenital aortic stenosis may be compatible with life for many years.

In the foregoing case, the cusps were filled with calcareous material and the valves constituted a collar of calcified material causing great narrowing of the aortic orifice. It is all the more remarkable that the deceased could live for 28 years and that he was able to engage in minor physical activities prior to his unexpected and sudden death.[8]

Sub-Aortic Stenosis

A 16-year-old seemingly healthy girl collapsed and died during a dance. Autopsy revealed the presence of a congenital subaortic stenosis, an open ductus arteriosus, and extreme hypertrophy of both ventricles. The stenotic lesion appeared as a firm raised fibrous ring of tissue below the base of the aortic valve. Up to the time of the fatal seizure there had been no signs or symptoms of the threatening catastrophe.

This is a rare case. In his survey of malformations of the heart, the experienced Arthur Keith[68] mentioned that he had seen only four cases. Mönckeberg[69] knew of only one case which he said is on view in the pathology collection of Tübingen University.

Sub-aortic stenosis, always a congenital anomaly, is caused by a ring of fibrous tissue situated approximately one centimeter below the aortic valves. It is caused by the persistence of a band or membrane of connective tissue immediately beneath the aortic valves.

Hypoplasia of the Arterial System

Immediately after an international rugby game at Johannesburg, South Africa, the 32-year-old captain of the Transvaal Team collapsed and died. At autopsy a hypertrophied heart weighing 482 g was found. All cardiac cavities were dilated. On histological examination, numerous fibrotic patches were seen irregularly distributed in the walls of the left ventricle. The aortic valve was competent. The mitral valve admitted two fingers.

The coronary artery tree was grossly underdeveloped. The left coronary artery showed numerous atheromatous areas. Below the orifice of the left coronary artery and at a point midway along the anterior descending branch the lumen was severely narrowed by atheromatous patches. The descending aorta was grossly hypoplastic measuring a little over half an inch in diameter, which is less than half the normal size. The enlarged spleen showed on section marked excess of lymphoid tissue. The small left kidney was the seat of advanced hydronephrosis. The left ureter was sharply kinked one inch above the bladder; the right kidney was hypertrophied.

There was a persistent thymus gland weighing 26 g (normal weight at this age, 15 g) containing numerous large Hassall's corpuscles presenting the picture of an active gland, rather than the involutionary organ which one would expect at the age of 32 years. Genital organs were conspicuously small. All lymphoid structures were hyperplastic, including those of the thorax, nasopharynx, intestinal canal, and the lymph node.

The propositus had been one of the most prominent South African rugby players of his time. He was known as "the iron man of rugby," had represented the country at home as well as in Britain, Australia, and New Zealand. An identical twin brother had drowned at the age of 30 years. The captain of the Springbok team supplied the following information:[70]

I have known L. since 1931, played on the same team with him on numerous occasions. During 1937 and 1938, I traveled with him to Australia and New Zealand. I always regarded L. as a very ill man. He used to complain of severe pain in the lower portion of his back, thought to be due to kidney trouble. On many occasions I massaged his back because of these pains. He also suffered from boils. At every football match he felt sick, used to put his finger into his throat until he vomited whereafter he felt better. Alcoholic drinks made him nauseous. His stamina had been exceptionally good until about two years prior to his death when his efficiency deteriorated. He had a husky voice, smoked heavily, and suffered from chronic bronchitis. His twin looked the same as L., had the same husky voice, and played the same type of game as his brother. In 1937 he drowned. His body was never found. During the three months preceding L.'s death he lost more than 20 lbs. in weight. A roentgenogram of his chest taken six months before he died did not show the cardiac hypertrophy seen at autopsy.

Hypoplasia of the arterial system is a possible cause of unexpected fatalities in association with exercise. The condition need not preclude top class athletic performance.[71] The issue was discussed in an editorial in *The Lancet* of February 22, 1969.[72] The mechanism of death during exertion in cases of the kind under reference is not fully understood.

Hypoplasia of the aorta, at times combined with hypoplasia of the entire arterial system, characterizes many kinds of congenital anomalies of the aortic valve and of the ascending aorta. The evidence obtained at autopsy of the foregoing case reminds one of the concept of a "Status Thymico-Lymphaticus" discussed by Palthauf of Vienna in 1889 and in 1890: "A lymphatic constitution distinguished by a persistent thymus gland, active Hassall's corpuscles, hypoplasia of the arterial system and abundant lymphatic tissue."[73,74]

An elaborate study of the status thymico-lymphaticus was published in 1945 by Jesse L. Carr.[75] It reviewed the historical background and consideration of normal thymic weight, experimental and clinical findings of status thymico-lymphaticus and causes of death in lymphatism. The paper is extensively illustrated and contains a number of autopsy reports, but this "status" is no longer accorded general recognition. (See also H.F. Otto. Pathologie des Thymus. Springer Verlag, Berlin, Heidelberg, 1984. pp. 298.)

Congenital Anomalies of Coronary Arteries

Normally the left coronary artery arises in the sinus of the left aortic cusp and subsequently divides into an anterior descending and a circumflex branch. The right coronary artery arises in the right aortic sinus and passes around the right ventricle to reach the right posterior portion of the heart. The right aortic sinus is called "anterior sinus" according to the *Basel Nomina Anatomica* (BNA) nomenclature of 1896, and "ventral sinus" according to the *Jena Nomina Anatomica* (NK) system of nomenclature of 1935. The nomenclature used in this chapter is the *Internationalia Nomina Anatomica* (INA) nomenclature of 1955.[76]

Fatal Collapse of School Boy

A 14-year-old high school student participated in a cross-country race of over two miles. After completing the contest, he walked to the dressing room nearby where he was found dead 20 minutes later. The boy had never been seriously ill. He was believed to be exceptionally fit since he belonged to the school's track team and walked or ran twice daily a distance of five miles between his home and school. A few days prior to his death he had passed a routine medical examination.[77]

At autopsy the heart weighed 350 g (normal cardiac weight of 190-225 g for boys of the same age). The enlargement was due to marked hypertrophy of the myocardium of the left ventricle. Both coronary arteries originated from a common funnel in the right aortic sinus. The lumen of the left branch was half the normal size. The course of the vessel led through the sulcus between the aorta and the pulmonary artery toward the anterior surface of the heart where it formed a siphon-type kink before dividing into its circumflex and anterior descending rami. The right coronary artery was of normal caliber and could be traced to its minute terminations.

Sections of the coronary artery failed to reveal atheromatous changes or other abnormalities. Histological examination of the myocardium yielded no evidence of recent or old infarction, no signs of acute or chronic myocarditis, and no scarring.

The reduction of blood flow through the anomalous left coronary artery had caused marked left ventricular hypertrophy, but did not render the heart incapable of complying with the demands of strenuous athletic exercise.

Normally, the entire coronary artery tree opens up during exercise at the same time. It is possible that being encased in the narrow sulcus between aorta and pulmonary artery, the left coronary artery was unable to expand while the right branch dilated normally. Thus, inequality of oxygen supply to the myocardium is thought to have ensued, producing electrical potential differences and death from ventricular fibrillation. The hypertrophy of the left ventricle must be assumed to have been progressive over the years. It is reasonable to imagine that the oxygen supply through the two differently sized branches of the coronary artery increased until it reached critical proportions during exercise.

The deceased had been able to indulge in strenuous activity for many years prior to the fatal episode.

Additional Case Descriptions [3,78]

The following are summaries of additional observations of our own and of observations reported by other authors of congenital abnormalities of coronary arteries in subjects who had died suddenly and unexpectedly in association with physical exertion.

An internationally known rugby player, 32 years of age, collapsed after a game and died within a few minutes. His autopsy revealed a generalized hypertrophied and dilated heart weighing 482 g. Lumina of coronary arteries and aorta were conspicuously small. The descending aorta measured $1/2$ inch in diameter, which is less than half the normal size. Microscopically several areas of myocardial fibrosis were found within the papillary muscles and at the base of the left ventricle.

A 27-year-old pneumatic drill operator died suddenly during work. The left coronary artery originated from the pulmonary artery. Origin and distribution of the right coronary artery were normal. Extensive degenerative changes were seen in the myocardium and in the papillary muscles.

A 24-year-old soldier died after a long distance race. The left coronary artery originated from the pulmonary artery. The circumflex branch was hypoplastic, measuring only two centimeters in length. Origin and course of the right coronary artery were normal. Its lumen was exceptionally wide. There were diffuse multiple fibrous patches in the myocardium but no inflammatory reaction was found.

A woman, 22 years of age, who had apparently been in perfect health, died suddenly while skipping rope after lunch. At autopsy no trace of the left coronary artery was found. The right coronary artery was of average size and the main blood supply to the left ventricle came from its descending branch. The greater part of the myocardium of the left ventricle was replaced by fibrous tissue.

An 11-year-old boy collapsed after running a quarter of a mile. He was dizzy, nauseated, and soon became cyanotic; this was followed by a generalized seizure. He was admitted to a hospital. Roentgenogram of the chest suggested pulmonary edema. Death occurred 19 hours after the syncope. At post-mortem examination the left coronary artery was seen to arise behind the right aortic valve and passed between the aorta and pulmonary artery. There was a fresh infarct involving the anterolateral and the anteroseptal portions of the subendocardial portions of the myocardium. Microscopic examination revealed areas of early degenerative changes, with loss of cross-striation and infiltration with neutrophils and histiocytes. This is the only case in the series with an interval of almost one day between collapse and death.

A 16-year-old high school basketball player collapsed during a game and died within a few minutes. At autopsy both coronary arteries were seen to arise from the right sinus of the aortic valve whose cusps appeared to have been rotated clockwise around the longitudinal axis of the aorta. A ring of connective tissue surrounded the proximal portion of the left coronary artery which passed through the sulcus between aorta and pulmonary artery. The right branch of the coronary artery turned dorsally and proceeded in an anteroposterior direction through the sulcus between aorta and superior vena cava. Microscopic examination failed to show pathologic changes of any kind in the coronary arteries or the myocardium.

In a 16-year-old boy who had suffered a myocardial infarction while running, Kimbiris, et al.[51] noticed that the left coronary artery originated from the right sinus of Valsalva. (This patient responded to conservative treatment and was discharged after five weeks.)

Virmani, et al. clarified the presumed mechanism of sudden death in subjects with congenital coronary artery anomalies. Of 22 patients who had died suddenly and whose autopsy failed to reveal significant anatomical causes of death other than the congenital anomalies of the coronary artery 59% had acute angle takeoff, 41% had ostial valve-like ridges. The authors hypothesized that aortic root dilation may compress coronary arteries with acute angle take-off and that ostial valve-like ridges may act as occlusion valves. "Either may cause acute obstruction of the coronary artery and lead to sudden death."[79]

Clarence DeMar

Not all congenital anomalies of the coronary arteries are of clinical relevance. A post-mortem examination was conducted on the famous long distance runner, Clarence DeMar, who died at the age of 70. He had participated in over 1,000 races, including 34 Boston marathon competitions of which he won seven. His last race at the age of 68 was undertaken despite the presence of a colostomy necessitated by a malignant tumor. Currens and White[12] reported that DeMar's coronary arteries were significantly large, "2 or 3 times the normal diameter."

The congenital anomaly of his coronary arteries undoubtedly facilitated the attainment of DeMar's extraordinary athletic achievements.

CARDIAC TUMORS

Mesothelioma

Wolf and Bing[80] reported the results of the autopsy of a man who had died suddenly after an Adam-Stoke attack: serial sectioning of the conduction system revealed a grey-white area measuring not more than 0.2 cm in length situated near the atrio-ventricular junction below the mitral valve in the interventricular septum of the heart. Serial sections showed the mass to be a "mesothelioma" which replaced the AV node and extended into the conduction system, proximal and distal to the node. The author writes that the minute lesion is the smallest tumor ever observed to cause sudden death.

By contrast, reference will be made to two observations of large intracardiac lesions that were for long periods asymptomatic. In one instance the tumor eventually caused a sudden and unexpected fatal seizure. Neither of them impinged upon the conduction system.

Fibroma

While playing at home, a 7-year-old girl collapsed and died within minutes. Prior to the fatal seizure the child had seemed to be healthy and physically fit. Autopsy revealed a chestnut-sized intracardiac mass attached to the left ventricle. Histologically the tumor, a "fibroma," was composed entirely of fibrous tissue.[81]

Hemangioendothelioma

A Weekly Clinico-Pathological Exercise at the Massachusetts General Hospital dealt with the case of a 15-year-old girl who had been admitted because of a murmur and a right ventricular mass that had been localized echocardiographically.[82] The patient was fit and presented no symptoms of functional relevance. Exploratory cardiotomy revealed the right ventricle partially replaced by a large mass involving the entire anterior wall and the outflow tract. It extended over the atrio-ventricular groove into the interventricular septum. The tumor was considered unresectable since excision would have required removal of the entire anterior portion of the right ventricle, the outflow tract and a portion of the interventricular septum. Examination of biopsied specimens showed fibrotic tissue containing vessels and entrapped myocytes. A reticulin stain confirmed the vascular nature of the tumor classified as capillary hemangionma or "hemangioendothelioma."

LESIONS OF CONDUCTION SYSTEM

For most functions of the heart its nerves are as important as its coronary arteries, but this is particularly true concerning cardiac rhythm, conduction and repolarization. It is thus paradoxical that postmortem correlative studies of sudden death virtually always include careful scrutiny of the coronary arteries but only rarely of the cardiac nerves or ganglia . . . Some cardioneuropathies are found in the absence of any other significant structural abnormality detect-

able in the heart and these are designated as a primary cardioneuropathies. A viral etiology or some heritable disorder must rank high among possible causes. Secondary cardioneuropathies are those observed in association with almost every disease that can affect the heart. (T.N. James[83])

In 1967 James[34] postulated that autopsies of young athletes who die suddenly require inclusion of serial sectioning of the conduction system. He subsequently presented additional evidence elaborating and substantiating the importance of his demand.

3 Case Reports by Thomas N. James

The post mortem findings of an 18-year-old youth who had died while playing football included the results of the histological examination of the sinus node artery which showed marked narrowing by a bizarre medial hyperplasia; at several points the arterial lumen was completely occluded by additional intimal proliferation.

A second case, also communicated by James pertained to a 15-year-old boy who had died while playing. Serial sections of the conduction system revealed microscopic foci of degeneration in the AV node and in the His bundle, as well as recent necroses with round cell infiltration. Close to the AV node the main sinus node artery was thickened, one of its major branches was nearly occluded by medial hyperplasia and intimal proliferation.

In 1980 James, et al.[85] detailed the results of examinations of serial sections of the cardiac conduction system of a 32-year-old man who died suddenly while driving. A tiny fibroma close to the His bundle; and small inflammatory foci adjacent to the sinus- and atrio-ventricular nodes were identified.

Bharati, et al.'s Cases[86]

Bharati, et al. described two cases of sudden death of young athletes in whom autopsy disclosed lesions involving the conduction system. The first was that of a 15-year-old boy who collapsed while playing soccer. He died 35 minutes later. The heart weighed 300 g. Histological examination revealed diffuse myocardial fibrosis; serial sections of the conduction system showed fatty infiltration and mononuclear cell infiltration of the sino-auricular and auricular-ventricular nodes.

Bharati, et al.'s second case concerned a 17-year-old boy who died during a football scrimmage. The heart weighed 355 g. The right ventricular walls were dilated and hypertrophied. Serial sections of the conduction system showed infiltration of mononuclear cells around the sino-auricular node, with fatty infiltration and fibrosis of the auricular-ventricular node. There was diapedesis of mononuclear cells into the penetrating portions of the AV bundle, and increase in collagen and elastic fibers and infiltration of inflammatory cells in the entire bundle of His.

Sudden Deaths in Three Generations

J.R. Green, et al.[87] studied a family in which ten instances of sudden death had occurred in three generations. In most instances syncopal episodes had preceded the terminal seizures. Among the fatalities was that of a 15-year-old boy who collapsed and died as he completed a 100-yard sprint in a school track meet. He had been examined two weeks earlier and no abnormalities were revealed. His 14-year-old sister collapsed and died on hearing of her brother's death. She was known to have experienced occasional syncopal episodes. At a recent medical examination, which included roentgen screening and ECG testing, she was declared normal. A year earlier a 10-year-old sister had fainted while walking on a beach and could not be resuscitated from ventricular fibrillation. She too had been examined and declared normal. Clinical studies on 22 surviving members of the family failed to reveal signs or symptoms of cardiac anomalies.

At the autopsy of the 15-year-old boy who had died after running, the nodal artery could not be identified in serial sections of the conduction system. At the autopsy of his sister histological examination revealed hypoplasia of the right bundle branch and spurious branches of both portions of the bundle of His.

The histological evidence obtained in the above mentioned two cases and the high frequency of fainting episodes preceding death in the family suggests that a non-sex-linked gene had produced the anatomical defects in the conduction system which were responsible for the fatalities.

Cardiac Aftermath of Athletic Trauma

An acute mechanized insult to a previously normal coronary artery circulation may result in transient myocardial ischemia or myocardial infarction. (D.S. Baim and D.C. Harrison[88]*)*

Cardiac injury caused by the application of blunt violence to the thorax falls into three groups: commotion, contusion and laceration. (Alan R. Moritz[89]*)*

COMMOTIO CORDIS

Tear of Right Ventricle

During a championship game, a 24-year-old soccer player stopped a ball with his chest. A few minutes later he left the field because of a burning substernal pain, collapsed and died within minutes.

Autopsy showed a tear two centimeters in length in the right ventricle. Histological examination revealed extensive scarification of the torn part of the myocardium as well as patches of endarteritis obliterans. Prior to the game the athlete's physical performance capacity had been unimpaired. As to the immediate cause of the fatal syncope the trauma plus the presence of endarteritis obliterans are noteworthy. The latter raises the question of a possible role of chronic myocarditis.[90]

A case of cardiac infarction in a football player after stopping a sharp ball with his chest was reported by Weber.[91] Schlomka[92] saw a tennis player collapse unconscious after being hit on the chest by a small ball during a tournament.

Review of Literature

Deutsch[93] reported a case of death in the boxing ring of a champion who had received a "hook" to the apical region of the heart. He was counted out and died on the spot. Autopsy revealed an enlarged heart with hypertrophy of the left ventricle. The aorta was hypoplastic, its circumference at the level of the diaphragm was 42 mm.

Jankovitch[94] reported the case of a boxer 21 years old who while running a temperature of 101°F participated in a boxing match. In the first round he received several blows to the heart region whereupon he collapsed and died within fifteen minutes. At autopsy a persistent thymus gland weighing 30 g was found, abundance of lymphatic tissue and a hypertrophic heart (370 g). Microscopic examination of myocardium revealed infiltration with leucocytes, monocytes and eosinophil cells.

Warburg[95] described the case of a policeman who fell ill after receiving a heavy blow on the chest and died 15 days later. Autopsy showed a fresh anterior wall infarct of the left ventricle. Sections of coronary arteries revealed advanced atherosclerosis; the main stem of the left coronary artery was completely obliterated by an embolus.

In reply to a question relating to myocardial infarction occurring in a 57-year-old man who had been struck over the precordium by a golf ball, Beck[96] concurred with the view that the precordial blow by the golf ball had bruised the heart. He added that the clinical manifestations of myocardial infarction and myocardial contusion may be so similar that differentiation becomes impossible.

Moullin[97] described a young football player who collapsed unconscious after receiving a blow over the sternum. He was cyanosed and his condition deteriorated the next day. Pericardiotomy was performed and two ounces of thin dark fluid were emptied.

While exercising, a 65-year-old man fell with his chest against a horizontal bar. He continued exercising but became ill after an hour. Five weeks later pericardiotomy was performed and 200 cc of blood were emptied. Four months later the patient died. Post-mortem study revealed a canal-like rupture of the right ventricle. A ventricular wall around the rupture showed advanced fatty infiltration. Coronary arteries and aorta were atherosclerotic.[98]

While playing softball, a young man was struck on the left side of the chest by the ball. He became ill during the ensuing night with substernal pains radiating into the left arm. Electrocardiogram confirmed the diagnosis coronary thrombosis. He died ten months later. Autopsy revealed the right coronary artery to be completely occluded. A healed infarction involved the lateral wall of the left ventricle, a recent infarction involved the lateral wall of the left ventricle, a recent infarction of the posterior wall. The right coronary artery showed advanced atherosclerosis.

Schlomka[99,100,101] conducted animal experiments which left no doubt that non-penetrating trauma to the chest can severely and permanently damage a previously normal heart. A diseased heart is especially vulnerable to commotio cordis.

Endocarditis After Athletic Trauma

A 17-year-old football player received a kick against his right hip.

Three days later he fell ill, became delirious, developed neck rigidity and signs of pneumonia, followed by acute endocarditis. During the ensuing two days his temperature rose to 106.6°F, and he died the next day. His mother reported that he had suffered from boils and attacks of sore throat. Autopsy revealed a hypertrophied left ventricle and a fresh large crumbling thrombotic mass protruding from the ventricular surface of the anterior curtain of the mitral valve. A small ruptured aneurysm attached to the valve was noted beneath the thrombus.[102]

Cerebral Embolism Following Contusion of the Heart

A 16-year-old school boy took part in a competitive boxing match. He received severe blows to the left side of the chest and "was in agony." The fight had to be stopped. Two hours later he suffered a sharp pain over his precordium. The next day he noticed that exercise brought on the pain. Two days later his left leg suddenly became dead below the hip and he felt very faint. Shortly afterwards he had a general convulsion followed by confusion and headache. On admission to the hospital the left leg was spastic, there was ankle clonus, tendon jerks were increased and there was an extensor plantar response. Voluntary movements were considerably impaired. A soft systolic murmur was heard over the mitral area together with a basal pericardial rub. The ECG revealed partial heart block with occasional omission of auricular systole as well as disturbance of AV conduction. An electroencephalogram taken the following week showed suppression of all waves in the parietal region.

A few months prior to the above episode the boy had been boxing at school and the fight had to be stopped in the first round as he was in severe pain following "concentrated punishment to the region of his heart." The pain continued for the next week and was aggravated by exercise. Presumably the boy's heart was bruised at this time and rendered more susceptible to subsequent damage. "It is impossible to escape the conclusion that the embolus was the direct result of the myocardial damage which was clearly demonstrated in the ECG, and that the actual cause of the embolus was a mural clot." (Parsons-Smith and Williams[103])

External Iliac Artery Thrombosis

A racing cyclist complained of a sharp pain in his left thigh and calf while walking. The pain passed off when he rested. He reported that when he was cycling the left leg quickly tired and the right leg was forced to do most of the pedalling. Oscillometer readings were reduced in the left leg. The femoral pulse was less marked on the left side. During an exercise tolerance test the patient complained of a feeling of discomfort in the left thigh. The left foot was paler than the right. A left external iliac artery thrombosis was diagnosed. The patient was operated on and an arteriectomy was performed. A thrombus was found extending from the division of the left common iliac artery to a point 1.25 cm below Poupart's ligament. The thrombosed segment was dissected free and excised. A left lumbar sympathectomy was also undertaken, the first three lumbar ganglia and intervening chain being removed. An arteriogram showed excellent collateral circulation. (Boyd and Jepson[104])

Traumatic Left Ventricular Aneurysm (Glancy, Yarnell and Roberts)[105]

A 20-year-old athlete was struck in the chest while playing football. A few minutes later severe substernal pain developed, followed after a month by intermittent claudication of the left calf and numbness, paralysis, and pain in both legs. The popliteal posterior tibial and dorsalis pedis arterial pulses were absent bilaterally. An ECG showed an anteroateral myocardial infarct. Claudication persisted. Twelve months later the patient played touch football but shortly afterwards noted numbness of both legs. Cine-angio-cardiography revealed an apical aneurysm. A cardiac operation was performed and a densely fibrotic area 2 x 22 cm of the left ventricular apical wall excised. Eight months later the patient was readmitted to hospital because of the sudden appearance of brain-stem infarction. A right vertebral arteriogram showed occlusion of the basilar artery. A variety of complications arose during the illness: inability to handle secretions necessitating tracheostomy; thrombosis at the site of the right brachial arteriotomy requiring thrombectomy; right femoral arterial embolization leading to embolectomy; recurrent cerebral emboli; and gastrointestinal hemorrhage requiring nine transfusions and cessation of heparin therapy. ECG was unchanged from that obtained after the trauma. Concomitant with the femoral arterial embolization and gastrointestinal bleeding, symptoms of acute inferior infarction appeared. The clinical picture of mesenteric arterial occlusion developed and the patient died.

At autopsy the left ventricular apex of the heart (wt 330 g) was found to be extensively scarred; a thrombus was attached to it. There was extensive scarring of the posterior left ventricular wall. The anterior descending coronary artery was severely narrowed nine centimeters from its origin by an organizing and fresh thrombus. The midline basilar portion of the pons was necrotic, and the basilar artery was occluded by thrombotic material. There was a fresh thrombus in the superior sagittal sinus and in the superior mesenteric artery five centimeters from its origin. The small intestine was distended and focally infarcted. Infarcts were found in kidneys and spleen; the right femoral artery was occluded by a recent thrombus.

Chapter III

COLLAPSE SYNDROMES

It is remarkable how seldom the physician or nurse observe brief, transient, alarming seizures, including syncope. I examined the hospital records of 230 patients suffering from attacks of various types of syncope, and found that in no case were the episodes observed by physicians or nurses. (Weiss[106])

Scope and Limitation of Autonomic Nervous Control

FATAL collapses associated with physical activity are triggered by acute breakdowns of autonomic control. During exercise the autonomic nervous system operates on a level of integration different from that on which it operates at rest. In respect of the former the term "heterostasis" was introduced in 1958.[107] It extends the concept of "homeostasis" relating to Claude Bernard's classical description in 1867 of "the constancy of the internal milieu."[108] Homeostasis characterizes the status of the autonomic nervous system at rest; heterostasis the sequelae of deployment of the autonomic nervous system during exercise.

The limitations of heterostatic control have been identified from analyses of a variety of collapse syndromes in athletes following strenuous muscular performances, each of them revealing a breakdown pattern of its own. With the exception of acute failure of termoregulation, the syndromes under review rarely have fatal consequences.

I have seen all collapse syndromes discussed in the ensuing chapter, experienced many of them myself during a long period of competing in national and international athletic contests and described them in a number of publications, some of them during my student years.*

HYPERTHERMIA (HEAT STROKE)

I am of the opinion that in healthy subjects the only serious potential risk to life from violent exercise is heat stroke — a danger well exhibited by examples I have seen of alarming collapse and, on one occasion, death. The correct precaution would be to prohibit the race in circumstances in which an occurrence might be expected — a moisture laden atmosphere, a following wind and the early afternoon of a day with a shade temperature of 85°F (29.5°C) or higher. (Sir Adolphe Abrahams[109])

Heat stroke should be suspected if a marathon is run on a warm day and a runner develops some of the following premonitory symptoms and signs. He may become irritable and aggressive and may even assault anyone who tries to remonstrate with him or help him; or he may display emotional instability with hysterical weeping or he may be apathetic and fail to respond to questioning. In this phase, the subject may be disoriented in time and space. He may run the wrong way around the track and be unaware of the time of day. He may develop an unsteady gait and a glassy stare. Finally he may collapse and become unconscious or he may have a convulsive seizure. His skin may be hot and dry or he may sweat profusely. His pulse may be rapid and feeble or it may be full and bounding. (C.H. Wyndham[110])

Dehydration (Sogar, et al.[111])

A 19-year-old farmer had been participating for three months in a physical training course demanding severe effort. In the last three days he had bloodless diarrhea, not accompanied by fever. He did not report sick, but decreased drastically food and fluid intake, believing this to be a remedy. On May 28, 1967, at 7 a.m., his team

*"Die Sportkrankheit" Klin Wschr 21:984-985, May 1930; "Zur Frage der Beurteilung von Herzfällen in der sportärztlichen Praxis." Med Klin 29:1070-1074, 1933; Zusammenbrüche beim Sport (Monograph). Manzsche Verlags und Universitäts-Buchhandlung, Wien, 1936; "Medical Problems of Aviation." J Roy Army Med Corps, London, 1939; "Syncope in Athletes (monograph)." Manpower, South African Government Publication, Vol 5-6(1-2):1-198, 1947; "Indisposition after Running" in International Research on Sport and Physical Education, Springfield, Thomas, 1964: 692-689; "Marked sinus and A-V nodal bradycardia with interference-dissociation in an athlete". J Sports Med Phys Fitness 9(2):128-129, 1969; "Altitude Diseases." New Engl J Med 280(25): 1420-1422, 1969; "8.90:Bob Beamon's World Record." Olympic Review, Lausanne, Nov/Dec 1972.

set out for an eight kilometer run. Even though his diarrhea was now arrested, the patient decided not to take food or drink before the run. (Meterologic measurements showed 24°C dry bulb and 20°C wet bulb.) At the end of the exercise, the patient became comatose. His rectal temperature was 41°C. He was at once sprinkled with water and given a saline infusion. The orderly and the physician who saw him several minutes after he lapsed into coma noted that he was sweating.

On admission to a hospital, at 9 a.m., the patient had a temperature of 40.7°C, pulse rate was 160 beats per minute, and blood pressure was 100/500 mm Hg. He was in deep coma with spastic extremities and in a state of excitation. Tendon reflexes were present; Babinski was negative. The skin was hot and sweating. Laboratory examinations disclosed the following values: sodium, 140 mEq/1; potassium, 4.1 mEq/1; chlorides, 108 mEq/1; carbon dioxide, 20.3 mEq/1; hemoglobin, 15.9 ggm/dl; and hematocrit, 58%. Catheterization yielded five ml of dark yellow urine ("machine-oil") containing protein (2 +), granular and hyaline casts, and leukocytes.

Cooling was begun immediately — with sponges soaked in ice-cold water, ice cubes, and ventilation — but the patient began to shiver and motor excitation increased to a point that cooling could not be continued, despite the administration of a "lytic cocktail" — chlorpromazine, 50 mg; promethazine hydrochloride (Phenergan), 25 mg; and meperidine (pethidine), 50 mg. When at 11 a.m. his rectal temperature was still 39°C, an infusion containing Thiopental Sidum (pentothal sodium) was given. The pulse rate was 132 beats per minute, and blood pressure rose to 95/70 mm Hg by noon. At 5 p.m. the patient awoke; his blood pressure was 120/80 mm Hg. At 7 and 11 p.m. he passed about 100 ml of dark, protein-containing urine. The patient slept well, and the next morning his temperature was normal and remained so throughout his hospital stay.

During the first day and the following days numerous investigations were performed in search of a possible infectious etiology: platelet counts started to decrease on the first day, and reached a minimum of 38,000/mm³ on the third day. Bleeding time was prolonged during the first four days. Petechiae and small hemorrhages were observed on the skin and the conjunctivae. Other clotting factors showed no abnormality. Serum glutamic oxaloacetic transaminase (SGOT) was forty units on admission, rose on the next day to 500, and reached a maximum of 1,350 on the fifth hospital day. On the sixth day the SGOT was 150; on the seventh, 90; and thereafter it reverted quickly to normal. The bilirubin level, 0.3 mg/dl on admission, rose rapidly to a maximum of 15 mg/dl on the sixth day, declined 1 mg/dl on the eighth day (on the seventh day dialysis was performed); and then continued to decrease. Lactic and dehydrogenase rose to 2,000 units. In the first 24 h, urine output was 320 ml with an urea content of 340 mg/dl. Blood urea, which was 48 mg/dl on admission, rose to 126 mg/dl the next morning. The picture was that of acute renal insufficiency with oliguria, low urea content of urine, and uremia. Hemodialysis was performed twice on the 7th and 12th day, then the blood urea level was 485 mg/dl and 525 mg/dl, respectively. The uremic stage was accompanied by clouded consciousness, recurrent melena, high serum phosphorus, and low serum calcium. Dialysis, already indicated on the fifth day, was delayed awaiting amelioration of the clotting and enzymatic disturbances. After the second dialysis, the urea decreased gradually and reverted to normal on the 25th day. Serum potassium, 4.1 mEq/1 on admission when the patient was severely dehydrated, decreased in the course of several hours to 3 mEq/1. Hyperkalemia did not appear throughout the disease, despite renal failure and repeated blood transfusions. The CO_2 was 20.3 mEq/1 on admission, decreasing to 18.1 mEq/1 the next day and to 15.3 mEq/1 on the third day. Thus, a state of hypokalemic metabolic acidosis was present. Follow-up examination after two months revealed normal findings. Blood urea was 33 to 39 mg/dl; specific gravity or urine, 1,022; and urea clearance, 58% of normal. Renal function studies performed one year following the heat stroke revealed normal glomerular filtration rate and renal plasma flow.

Cerebral Hemorrhage (Shibolet, et al.[112])

A previously healthy 21-year-old male set out on a march on 16 September 1964. On the previous day, which was a religious holiday, he did not drink nor eat. At noon he was seen to lag behind his comrades. Shortly afterwards, he lost consciousness. Half an hour later his underwear was noted to be wet. Several participants in the same

march complained of thirst and disorderly behavior. On admission
to the nearest hospital, about seven hours after losing consciousness,
he was in a coma, the skin was observed to be "rather dry," rectal
temperature was 38.9°C, pulse was 120, blood pressure was 70/50.
Laboratory investigations showed: hemoglobin, 22.9 g/dl blood;
leukocytes, 20,000/cubic ml blood; urea, 90 mg/dl blood; NA, 139
mEq/1; K, 6.2 mEq/1; serum glutamic oxaloacetic transaminase
(SGOT) 120 U; serum glutamic pyruvic transaminase (SGPT), 120
U: serum glutamic pyruvic transaminase (SGPT), 45 U. During the
night, 3,000 ml of saline were administered intravenously. Blood
pressure rose to 120/80 and 160/100; however, the patient's state of
consciousness did not improve. Lumbar puncture revealed a clear
spinal fluid under normal pressure containing 87 mg protein/dl.
Until noon on the day after admission, the patient excreted 500 cc of
urine containing many granular cylinders with 3 + reaction for protein. When the blood urea rose to 130 mg/dl blood, the patient was
transferred to another hospital.

On admission, 18 September 1964, he was semi-conscious, react-
ing only to painful stimuli, and was sometimes able to obey simple
orders. A small conjunctival hemorrhage was seen in the left eye.
General hyperreflexia was present. Rectal temperature was 37.6°C;
pulse, 88; blood pressure 150/110; respirations 20/min. Lumbar
puncture revealed bloody xanthochromic spinal fluid with 100 mg
protein/dl, and 21 white cells/cubic ml. The salient laboratory findings revealed the presence of renal failure, hepatic damage, and low
prothrombin levels, especially a decrease in clotting factor VII. The
patient was treated with intravenous fluid replacement, fresh plasma
and broad spectrum antibiotics (Kanamycin and penicillin). A tracheostomy was performed when respiratory difficulties and periods
of Cheyne-Stokes respiration appeared. X-rays of the chest, performed when purulent discharge appeared at the tracheostomy, revealed bilateral lung infiltrations, more prominent at the bases. On
the fifth day of illness, the patient died after sudden apnea, probably
as a result of damage to the central nervous system.

On post-mortem examination, the brain displayed a large hemorrhagic mass in the right cerebellum with destruction of brain tissue. A smaller punctate hemorrhage, 12 mm in diameter, was
present in the left occipital lobe. Microscopic examination showed

many cortical and subcortical hemorrhages. Microscopic clots, plugging the capillaries, were present at several sites in the cerebrum and cerebellum. Some large hemorrhages were present in the colon. In the left kidney there was a fresh infarct involving the renal cortex. Several degenerated tubules were filled with orange-brown cylinders. Widespread broncho-pneumonia was present in both lungs. The liver showed central lobular congestion.

Nephropathy Associated with Heart Stress and Exercise (Schrier, et al.[113])

> *Renal failure is seen in approximately ten percent of patients with heat stroke. Renal dysfunction also is common in patients with exertion in the absence of heat stroke. (Kevin T. Parsons, et al.[114])*

A 22-year-old man collapsed during a military training exercise held on a moderately warm day (outside temperature, 77°F). During the preceding days temperature had been in the middle 80's and humidity had been high. Immediately after the collapse, the patient's skin was hot and dry, his rectal temperature 108°F. A "grand mal" seizure occurred within the next hour. On transfer to a hospital blood pressure was 90/70 mm Hg. Initial laboratory data were as follows: hematocrit, 50m/11m; hemoglobin, 16.1 g/11 ml; BUN, 22.5 g/11 ml; and total carbon dioxide, 23 mEq/1. Urinalysis showed proteinuria, many red blood cells, and coarse granular casts. During the first twenty-four hours of hospitalization urine output was only 225 ml in spite of a total fluid intake of 3,600 ml and three trials with 12.5 mannitol intravenously. On the third hospital day intramuscular penicillin was given due to the suspicion of pneumonia. Oliguria persisted; the patient's mental status deteriorated; jaundice developed; BUN was 66 mg/100 ml serum potassium, 5.9 mEq/1, and total carbon dioxide of 9 mEq/1. Liver function tests were markedly abnormal; total bilirubin, 19.5 mg/100 ml; alkaline phosphatase, 17.6 King-Armstrong U: SGOT, 1,070 U; and cephalin flocculation, 4+. Platelet count of 80,000 was accompanied by a prolonged prothrobin time. On the ninth hospital day the patient died.

An autopsy of the lungs showed pulmonary congestion and edema with an early bronchopneumonia in both lower lobes. A focal area of subendocardial hemorrhage was found in the right ventricle of the heart. Diffuse central and midzonal degeneration of hepatic parenchymal cells was present. The cerebral cortex and the basal ganglia showed marked hyperemia without neuronal degeneration. Focal vacuolization and degeneration of skeletal muscle were present. The cerebral cortex and the basal ganglia showed marked hyperemia without neuronal degeneration. Focal vacuolization and degeneration of skeletal muscle were present. The right and left kidneys weighed 380 and 340 g respectively. Microscopically, the glomeruli, the larger vessels, and the interstitium were unremarkable. In both cortical and medullary regions numerous pigmented granular casts were observed in distal tubules and collecting ducts. Similar casts were present in many atrophic unidentifiable tubules in the cortex and in thin loops of Henle in the medulla. Because of postmortem alterations, unequivocal areas of tubular necrosis were not identifiable. Many peritubular capillaries contained collections of mononuclear cells and were severely congested.

Endotoxic Shock

Graber, et al.[115] described a case of fatal heat stroke in an athlete which was complicated by shock, septicemia, anuria, and coagulopathy. The patient who had recently undergone a wisdom tooth extraction developed endotoxemia, hypocomplementemia, hypoimmunoglobulinemia, and elevated serum lysozyme. Autopsy findings were consistent with those seen in experimental endotoxic shock and were characterized by numerous fibrin thrombi in arterioles. Blood cultures grew a predominance of *Providencia alcalifaciens. Klebsiella pneumoniae* was recovered from the antemortem flood culture, Proteus species from the autopsy blood. *P. alcalifaciens* grew from the autopsy lung tissue.

The authors consider the advisability of performing the Limulus lysate test for the determination of serum endotoxin levels in all cases of heat stroke to obtain information about the clinical course of such patients and to elucidate the role of circulating endotoxin as a potential fatal mechanism.

HYPOTHERMIA

Channel swimmers have thicker skinfolds, indicating more subcutaneous fat than is found in the average individual. When energy expenditure is high, an extra one mm. of subcutaneous fat thickness is equivalent to raising the temperature of the water surrounding the swimmer by as much as 1.5°C. The swimmer's greater thickness of subcutaneous fat plays an important role in preventing the development of hypothermia. Weight gains of 7-14 kg. in one season are common among Channel swimmers, some of whom put on weight purposely in training in order to withstand the cold. However, channel swimmers' total body fat, predicted from standard height-weight tables is far below average because of a proportionately greater muscular development. (LGCE Pugh[116])

While fatness is generally incompatible with fitness, channel swimmers are both fat and fit. (Pugh and Edholm[117])

How can channel swimmers swim for 12-22 hours and longer in water at a temperature of about 60°F (15.5°C) when shipwrecked persons survive in water at this temperature only four to six hours? A study by Pugh and Edholm yielded significant information on the puzzle.[117]

Long distance swimmers are distinguished by a singularly effective thermal insulation. Their physiques differ from those of other athletes in that they are fat as well as muscular. Channel swimmers' subcutaneous fat deposit amounts to twenty percent and more of their total body weight as against between two and five percent or less for long distance runners, skiers, cyclists, etc.

Fat is three times as good an insulator against heat loss as muscle. Unless a man is fat he cannot take up long distance swimming because he is unable to endure the cold water. Since the extra heat engendered by swimming is produced in the muscles, the difference between internal body temperature and water temperature increases with the result that the effectiveness of body fat as an insulator against heat loss is enhanced.

A series of tests was conducted with the Egyptian channel swimmer, J. Zirganos, and with Dr. Pugh, a former member of the 1953 British Himalaya Expedition. Zirganos was fat, Pugh thin. At the end of a swim of seven hours at a water temperature of 60.8°F (16°C), Zirganos' internal body temperature had remained unchanged; while Pugh began to shiver after swimming for twenty minutes. Ten minutes later he had to be lifted out of the water. His core body temperature had dropped from 99.5°F (37.5°C) to 92.7°F (35.8°C).

When the two men were tested as they lay motionless in cold

water, sharp decreases in internal body temperature occurred in both. During swimming Pugh showed a still greater loss of body heat while Zirganos' temperature rose or remained unaltered when he swam for many hours. Most people feel comfortable at skin temperature levels of 92.3°F (33.5°-24°C); Mr. Zirganos was at ease at skin temperatures as low as 86.0°-87.8°F (30°-31°C).

Antonio Albertondo of Argentina swam the English Channel both ways non-stop. He covered the distance in a little over forty-three hours. Water temperature was 62°F, 18° below that of the Parana River between Argentina and Paraguay in which he had previously completed a swim of 257 miles downstream in eighty hours. Before the double Channel crossing, he ate nothing. During the swim he asked for sandwiches, fruit and chicken broth. When he was within sight of the landing beaches of St. Margaret's Bay he began to falter saying, "I am cold." It took him two hours to do the last mile. At that time he was in a state of confusion, dazed, listless and sore. Towards the end of the swim he became lightheaded, heard weird sounds and imagined that the sea was filled with hundreds of dogs swimming with him.

Disturbances of consciousness due to the cold in long distance swimmers are not uncommon. In 1946 the Egyptian channel swimmer, Hamad, had to be taken out of the water after seven hours because he was in a confused state. In 1951 he was thirty-five pounds heavier and completed the channel crossing. One swimmer was unconscious for three hours after being removed from the race after being in the water for seven hours. On wading ashore the winner of the Ladies Channel Swim in 1951 had hallucinations; she saw animals all over the water.

DEATH FROM EXPOSURE

Death from exposure is the coroner's usual verdict when a hill walker or climber is found dead by a search party and there are no injuries to account for death. Cases occur every year in the hilly regions of Britain, but are seldom reported except in the popular press. It seems safe to assume that hypothermia is the cause of death in these cases, though there is no proof of this. Accidental hypothermia also occurs among potholers, yachtsmen, and dinghy sailors as a result of immersion in cold water. (LGCE Pugh[116])

Case Reports

A 19-year-old student entered the popular Four Inns Walk, a walking competition held annually in England. The course involves a forty-four mile walk over the moors at altitudes involving a total ascent and descent of 4,500 feet. Competitors usually take from 10 to 22 hours to complete the walk. On the day of the competition temperatures ranged from 3° to 7°C with winds up to 35 knots. The student who had a severe attack of influenza three weeks previously had taken part in the Four Inns Walk on two former occasions. The following is an excerpt of the official report presented by Pugh:

> G.W. began to flag around midday after the long climb to Bleaklow (2,000 ft) which they all found very tiring. By this time he had been out some 5½ hours, and had covered 12 miles. He was wet and cold, began to fall down frequently and his companions had to walk one on each side of him. Shortly afterwards, they sat down and one of them went for help which arrived within 2 hours. G.W. was then conscious and able to walk with assistance. At about 4:15 p.m. a rescuer stated that he was semiconscious and incoherent. By this time he was being carried by 3 rescuers. While they were carrying him along a narrow steep slope, he had a convulsion which threw the rescuers off their balance, and one of them fell 20 feet and hurt his chest. Eventually they were met by a stretcher party, and G.W. was carried on the stretcher in a thick kapok sleeping bag with waterproof cover. It was reported that on arrival at Alport Farm at 7:15 p.m., G.W.'s body was rigid and he had become very pale. A pulse was detectable at his temple. It was not stated whether he was conscious or not. One hour later at 8:15 p.m., he was admitted to Glossop Hospital, apparently dead. Artificial respiration and oxygen were given for 3 hours without success. (L.G. Pugh[116])

Necropsy revealed abrasions of knees and wrists. Lungs, liver and kidneys were congested. Heart was enlarged and congested; right ventricle distended and wall thinned out. Cause of death: acute myocardial failure after extreme exposure to cold. The pathologist thought that the attack of influenza might have contributed.

Two students (J.B. and M.W.) both aged 21 were experienced

hikers. M.W. had taken part in the Four Inns Walk in 1962. A third member of the team, R.K., gave evidence at the inquest.

The team started at 7:45 a.m. near Bleaklow. J.B. complained of cramps and kept stopping. He was going more and more slowly. They were all very wet; at this stage they lost their way and went about one mile off course. The time was not stated but it was probably early afternoon. J.B. became unsteady and his companions had to urge him on. In the words of R.K.: "J.B. was slowly tiring and getting unsteady. We had to help him although I was not much good because I was stumbling too." They helped him by walking on each side. He did not say much, but when he did speak his voice was normal. When he could go no further they sat down, and M.W., who was the fittest went to reconnoitre. When R.K. went to fetch help, M.W. stayed with J.B. R.K. met a rescue party and was assisted down to Alport Farm, suffering from exposure. Two parties searched for M.W. and J.B. but failed to find them.

It is thought M.W. may have stayed with J.B. until he died, and started back perhaps in the dark, when his torch may have given out. Their bodies were found two days later. J.B.'s body was in a stream bed, partly in the water. M.W.'s body was lying covered with snow about one mile to the west.

Necropsy findings were essentially similar to those obtained in the foregoing case except that the organs were less congested.

ORTHOSTATIC COLLAPSE

It certainly was a bold enterprise of nature to create quadrupeds like man or the giraffe with a predominantly vertical extension, who carry their heads and hearts at a considerable distance above the center of gravity of the body. (O. Gauer and H. Thron[118])

Historical Review

Von Humboldt[119] saw fainting spells during his mountaineering expedition in South America. Mosso[120] gave a detailed account of a vasomotor collapse affecting a soldier named Camozzi who indulged in dumbbell exercises on top of the Monte Rose (12,000 feet). Paul Bert[121] was the first to produce at will dizziness, muscular weakness and unconsciousness in healthy subjects in his low pressure chamber. In 1938 Henderson[122] wrote that he had seen many who were perfectly acclimatized to an altitude of 6,000 feet but who became sick when travelling by rail to Pike's Peak which is 14,000 feet high. "Many more collapsed unconscious after making the ascent on foot."

Sir Thomas Lewis[123] mentioned "fainting" as a "not infrequent symptom" of the "effort syndrome," a diagnostic entity that is no longer recognized. He stated that attacks occur often in patients exercising under emotional stress. He described the following case of a young soldier who had previously collapsed while saluting on guard duty.

> He began to feel queer as though his 'stomach had turned upside down.' He became dizzy. Pallor was noticed. His head fell forward on his knees. He was at once placed in a long easy chair and further observed. By this time pallor was intense and he was restless. The pulse was imperceptible, the heart sounds were distant, the rate of beating being 50 per minute. The action was for the most part regular. From time to time there were wretching movements, the pupils were little, if at all, dilated. He was limp, mentally confused and actually unconscious for several minutes. A heavy sweat broke out over the forehead, and spread over the chest and body. The pallor remained extreme. Respiration was slow and sighing. The pulse was imperceptible for several minutes . . . He was shakey and exhausted for 36 hours subsequently. (T. Lewis[123])

Orthostatic syncope in athletes almost invariably occurs after rather than during, exercise. Athletes are often more susceptible to fainting than non-athletes because of the vagotonic preponderance that characterizes the trained state, a fact of special importance to aviation medicine to which I have drawn attention in a paper in the *Journal of the Royal Army Medical Corps* in 1939.[124] Infection, fatigue, lack of food, warm environment, and altitude facilitate the onset of orthostatic syncope.

Chief symptoms of impending orthostatic collapse after athletic competitions are extreme breathlessness — at Mexico City accompanied by cyanosis of lips and nose, rarely encountered at sea level; a sharp fall of arterial blood pressure, extreme tachycardia and tachypnoea, accompanied by a feeling of helplessness or fear. If after exertion athletes stand motionless they are likely to faint. In Mexico City Galina Prosumentchikova fainted during the victory ceremony following the 100 m breaststroke final; John Ferris likewise collapsed on the victory stand after the 100 m butterfly final, both during the playing of the national anthems.

M. Burger[125] reported that after a marathon race runners responded to the Valsalva test with significantly greater fall of blood pressure than they did before the race.

Rook[126] wrote that women applicants for pilots' licenses should always be questioned for symptoms of giddiness occurring about the time of their periods.

The vagotonic shift predisposes to vaso-vagal 'overshoot': during the Ice Hockey World Championships held in Davos, Switzerland in 1931 I took blood samples from the Canadian National Team. When during the last intermission of the final game I withdrew blood from the cubital vein of one of the players, three team members fainted when they saw the blood spurting from the needle. The intermission had to be extended to enable the victims to recover. (Fortunately the Canadians won.)

During the 1928 Olympic Games, F. Deutsch[127] measured cardiac size in athletes before and after competitions. A marked decrease of end-diastolic volume was seen following exercise. He referred to the phenomenon as 'deminutio cordis'. Deutsch correctly interpreted his findings by explaining that during activity peripheral blood vessels dilate and that blood accumulates in the dependent part of the body while the subject stands. The filling of the heart is thus temporarily reduced.

Otto Gauer[118] has comprehensively discussed the "Postural Changes in Circulation". A deminutio cordis after exercise, he writes, does not occur if the subject is placed in the supine position. In 1972 Gauer, et al.[128] presented roentgenological evidence on the change of heart size in relation to posture and immersion in water. In one subject cardiac volume while standing was 689 ml; supine 771 ml; after immersion 922 ml. Jokl[129] showed that in competitive swimming the decline of speed with distance is much greater in running than in swimming: The heart of swimmers operates in a state of weightlessness, it need not work against gravity. Orthostatic collapses of swimmers in the water are not known.

If healthy young men can develop circulatory failure while standing erect after exercise, one may guess that similar circulatory changes may be readily induced in the older age groups, more severe in their manifestations and capable of serious consequences. (L.W. Eichna, S.M. Horvath and W.B. Bean[130])

A controlled study of post-exertional orthostatic hypotension was conducted by Eichna, Horvath, and Bean[130] who examined 33 young healthy soldiers at Fort Knox, Kentucky. Three exercise tests were applied: the pack test, the treadmill test, the hike, and endurance test. After the tests the subjects were examined on a tilt table whose position was changed alternately from erect to flat, and from flat to erect at five minute intervals. Heart rate and blood pressure were determined during the tests.

The post-exertional orthostatic responses were divided into three groups: syncopal, abnormal, and normal. The syncopal group included those subjects who developed syncope and were unable to remain erect for five minutes during either one or both of the two required erect periods after exercise. While erect their blood pressure was usually very low and their heart rate rapid but collapse rather than any level of blood pressure or heart rate was the criterion for inclusion in this category. When upright, these subjects developed the typical symptoms and signs of syncope, either singly or in varying combinations and intensity.

Almost invariably present were marked fatigue, drowsiness, apprehensiveness, increasing discomfort, nausea, abdominal cramps, lightheadedness and dizziness, and the sensation of impending collapse. In the more severe instances, dimness of vision progressing to tubular vision and "blackout", vomiting, disorientation, inability to move or obey commands even though failure to respond to them progressed to complete loss of consciousness and crumpling at the knees.

In approximately one-half of the subjects, orthostatic hypotension developed; in fifty percent, syncope resulted.

One soldier while standing erect following the Harvard Pack Test suffered a syncopal attack during which a *cardiac arrest for nineteen seconds* occurred.

A. Schlesinger[131] reported a like reaction to a fitness test of a healthy 35-year-old man after an ergospirometric examination. A "vagal reaction" appeared immediately after the test, manifested by pallor, cold sweating, nausea, bradycardia, and hypotension. The patient's condition deteriorated rapidly; he collapsed followed by *cardiac standstill*. Brisk chest thumping restored sinus rhythm and the patient regained consciousness. After five minutes of rest in a supine position he recovered completely.

Biggs [132] showed that normal subjects when raised quickly from a recumbent to an erect position react with a decline in cerebral blood flow; Lennox, et al. [133] reported that the oxygen content of the blood in the internal jugular vein is greatly reduced during the period of approaching unconsciousness.

VALSALVA PHENOMENON

Several years ago, I discovered and have since shown to my friends that I could interrupt at will my arteries by hindering the air from entering into my chest which I was at the same time compressing . . .

The cessation of the beat of the heart is immediately accompanied by that of the auricular and ventricular sounds and of the aortic and pulmonary murmurs. One still feels 3 to 5 very feeble pulsations and then there is a sudden cessation.

One day, when I held my breath a little longer than usual, I lost consciousness. While I was in this state, my assistants noted some convulsive movements of my face; when I returned to myself I had lost the memory of what had passed and for the first moment I could not recall where I was although my pulse had become palpable. I have kept in mind to desist from thoracic compression as soon as I felt fainting coming on and it is probable that if I should not do so, it would be dangerous for me and my life might perhaps be jeopardized. (E.F. Weber [134])

Expiratory effort against resistance with the closed glottis represents one of the greatest physiologic stresses to which the heart can be submitted. The diffusion of oxygen through the lung is suspended, oxygen saturation of the blood decreases most rapidly after exercise when oxygen requirements of the tissues are raised. The elevated intrathoracic pressure inhibits the return of blood to the heart causing an increase of venous pressure. The diminished output of the right ventricle thus caused as well as the increased intrapulmonary pressure interfere with the pulmonary circulation, with the result that the left ventricle is virtually empty. Filling of, and pressure in the ascending aorta decrease, and coronary blood flow diminishes sharply. Visscher[135] has commented on "the pressure gradient mechanism" on which coronary blood flow depends. "This pressure gradient," he wrote, "is measured by the difference in pressure between aorta, coronary sinus and right ventricle."

Loss of consciousness during weight lifting is a phenomenon with which competitiors are familiar. Compton, et al.[136] who measured introthoracic pressures during lifting obtained pressures as high as 260 mm Hg. Most contestants over-breathe before lifting with the result that the hyperventilation lowers expiratory carbon-dioxide levels. "Weight-lifters' blackout can be attributed to the reduced cardiac output and cerebral blood-flow associated with the Valsalva manoeuvre."

Bürger[127] devised a test to assess the effect upon blood pressure of blowing against a mercury column. Many healthy young men collapsed during the "Valsalva tests." Most were deeply unconscious; in several instances Bürger observed clonic cramps. Assumption of the horizontal position restored consciousness. The "Valsalva Collapse," Bürger wrote,[137] does not always involve loss of consciousness; sometimes only "the subject's knees give in." Loss of consciousness occurred most frequently when expiratory pressure was raised rapidly.

Swimming accidents may be due to unconscious performance of the Valsalva experiment:

H.S., 26 years old, swimmer, while bathing in a familiar place, sank suddenly. He was rescued, regained consciousness in a hospital. Of the accident and its cause he remembered nothing. He was tested a few days later, collapsed unconscious when blowing against a mercury column resistance of 50 mm Hg.

Albert B. Craig[138] has drawn attention to the fact that hyperventilation before breath-holding and exercise may delay the onset of urge to breathe and the situation thus engendered is of importance for an understanding of loss of consciousness during underwater swimming.

EFFORT MIGRAINE

Over the oxygen supply of the body, carbon dioxide spreads its protective wings. (F. Miescher)

"Effort migraine," or "effort sickness" is a fairly common occurrence among athletes. At competitions at sea level it is less frequent than at altitude. At the 1960 Olympic Games Congress in Rome, I discussed the similarity of effort migraine and acute altitude sickness.

Historical Review[139]

Symptomatologically, "effort sickness" is indistinguishable from "acute mountain sickness." Mild physical exertion at high altitudes causes attacks as severe as violent exertion does at sea level.

The history of the condition is interesting. In 1590, J. de Acosta,[140] a Jesuit priest, reported that he had become afflicted by severe nausea while riding on a donkey at an altitude of 17,500 feet in Peru. He interpreted his discomfiture rightly as having been due to the "rarified mountain air." In 1788, H.G. Saussure who ascended the Mont Blanc in Switzerland on foot observed that physical exertion may lead to "mountain sickness" at altitudes below 17,500 feet. In accordance with Lavoisier's demonstration in 1786 that life depends upon the availability of oxygen he theorized that "mountain sickness" ensues as the result of reduced oxygen pressure interfering with "the vital functions of the body." In 1814, Alexander von Humboldt noted during his South American travels that a trumpet blower became indisposed when he tried to play a tune at 12,000 feet; that the carriers serving with his mountain expeditions were particularly susceptible; and that physically trained subjects were more resistant to the strain of climbing at great heights. He also drew attention to the fact that signs and symptoms of "mountain sickness" invariably disappear during the descent.

Around the end of the nineteenth century, plans were drawn up to build a railway to the summit of Pike's Peak in Colorado, also one to the summit of Oroya in Peru, of Antofagasta in Chile, and of the Jungfrau in Switzerland, all of them situated at altitudes between 13,600 and 16,000 feet. Since the companies contemplating these costly engineering ventures wanted to be assured that prospective travelers would not be incapacitated by "mountain sickness," a number of scientific studies were undertaken to clarify issues. In 1903, the Swiss physiologist, H. Kronecker,[141] reported that "symptoms identical with those of 'mountain sickness' occur in athletes who compete in cycling, rowing and running races at sea level."

His findings were elaborated in 1960 by N. Zuntz, A. Loewy, Franz Müller, and W. Caspari[142] who summarized their observations as follows:

> The symptoms of physical exhaustion after maximal athletic performances at sea level may be analogous to those experienced by mountaineers at 12,000 feet and above. The cause of the bodily disturbance is in both instances the same: lack of oxygen ("anoxia") caused by the increased metabolic requirements brought about by muscular effort; or by the lowered oxygen tension in the atmospheric air.

In 1899 the Italian physiologist, A. Mosso,[120] discovered that loss of CO_2 is involved in "mountain sickness." He introduced the concept of "acapnia," i.e., deprivation of the body's CO_2 stores due to hyperventilation.

In 1911 Yandell Henderson[122] of Yale University organized a research expedition to the summit of Pike's Peak to study the changes attending transportation by train from sea level to an altitude of 12,100 feet. He was accompanied by three distinguished physiologists, viz., E.C. Schneider, C.G. Douglas and J.S. Haldane,[143] the latter two from England. They showed that by causing hyperventilation the diminishing oxygen pressure of the atmospheric air at high altitudes engenders a continuous loss of carbon dioxide. Thus altitude not only induces anoxia but also causes acapnia. Carbon dioxide is the physiological stimulus for breathing. Its disappearance removes the most important mediator of respiratory adjustment. "Acapnia," Henderson summarized, "is a deficiency of carbon dioxide that leads in turn to a deficiency of oxygen." This is one of the reasons why acute "mountain sickness" as well as "effort sickness" do not occur immediately following strenuous physical effort but only after an interval of several minutes. Some athletes "become sick" before a race or game when the psychological tension triggers off hyperventilation.

The study of "mountain sickness" and of "effort sickness" has lent new emphasis to the statement made in 1885 by the Swiss physiologist, F. Miescher:[143] "Over the oxygen supply of the body, carbon dioxide spreads its protecting wings."

The conclusion that uncomplicated "effort sickness" always has favorable prognosis does not necessarily apply in reference to its occurrence at high altitudes. In 1960 Charles S. Houston[144] of Aspen, Colorado gave an account of observations of collapses due to acute cardiac failure in previously healthy young men who during a cross country ski trip from Aspen carried packs weighing fifty pounds over a 12,000 foot pass in deep snow and cold weather. Similar cases have since been described in the medical literature, some of them with fatal outcomes.

The combination of high altitude and maximal physical effort may overtax the adaptive resources of the healthy human organism.

During the Olympic Games at Mexico City in 1968 the combination of reduced atmospheric pressure and exhaustive effort caused an unusually large number of athletes to be afflicted with the syndrome with all its classical manifestations: negative or scintillating scotoma, nausea, vomiting, and severe throbbing headache. *

D.J. Dalessio on Migraine

In the April 1974 issue of the journal, *Headache*, Donald J. Dalessio[145] devoted an editorial article to the syndrome described by me in 1930, quoting my original account:

> During my freshman year in medical school I ran as anchor-man in the mile relay team of my university in the German track championships in Jena, Thuringia. We won by the smallest possible margin. I was then seventeen years old and this was the first time I had been clocked in under fifty seconds. A few minutes after the race my happiness over the victory was interrupted by an attack of nausea, headache, prolonged weakness and vomiting. It lasted fifteen minutes whereupon it quickly subsided. None of my professors was able to explain the episode, nor could I find appropriate references in any textbook of physiology or medicine. (E. Jokl[146])

Appenzeller[147] has described altitude headache. He finds that headache is a prominent symptom of acute mountain sickness, and that it occurs almost universally above 12,000 feet for those not acclimatized to altitude. The headache is typically throbbing, often generalized, and aggravated by jolts, coughing or straining, suggest-

---

*For a comprehensive treatment of the subject, see: Jokl E., Jokl P.: "Exercise and Altitude." *Medicine and Sport*, Vol 1. Basel, Karger, 1968.

ing intracranial as well as extracranial vasodilation. The headache may not appear until six hours after attaining high altitude. It is not the immediate result of hypoxia, and does not respond quickly to oxygen. It seems likely that the symptoms are related to vasodilation, brain edema, and anoxia, and some diuretic agents have proved helpful in this situation.

"Mountain Sickness"

I believe that the term "acute mountain sickness" requires specifications, that in highly trained athletes altitude intensifies acute manifestations during or immediately after extreme competitive effort; that distinction between adequate and inadequate adaptation of altitude is important; that mountain sickness may be related to other altitude-induced disorders, some of which are modifiable by drugs; and that the susceptibility of athletes to infections at altitude is worthy of mention in this context. (See p. 68 ff.)

The term "acute mountain sickness" is used for different conditions. A. Loewy[148] included short lasting effort syndromes after exercise at altitude among the manifestations of "Bergkrankheit." In the chapter, "High Altitude Sickness" in Loeb's *Textbook of Medicine,* Robert C. Darling[149] writes that acute altitude sickness or acute mountain sickness occurs after a few hours exposure to elevations high enough to cause marked hypoxia. A.S. Forwand, et al.[150] confined their observations to a period of 40 hours after transportation of a group of young men to 12,800 feet, whereas Singh, et al.[151] extended their studies of acute mountain sickness over a period of several weeks.[139]

Seelinger, et al.[152] reported on a 26-year-old man who after running one and a half miles developed visual disturbances in the right field of vision and left-sided clumsiness associated with left frontal headache, pain over his left eye, nausea and vomiting. Examination of the visual fields showed a right superior quadrantic field defect, the electroencephalogram a left posterior temporal slow focus. The headache whose intensity had a tendency to fluctuate between exacerbation and remissions lasted for seven hours. Ergot had no effect. EMI scan revealed an infarct in the left occipital pole.

Robert G. Miller[153] described episodes of transient focal cerebral ischemia in a 32-year-old athlete who competed in a three mile run and a half mile swim. Less than an hour later he noted that his left arm and the left side of his face were numb and that his speech had become slurred. A mild, dull aching sensation appeared in the left temple within the next hour or two. The only neurologic abnormalities were slowing of rapid movements in the left hand (the patient was left handed), dysesthesia in the left arm, mild weakness of the extensor of the left great toe, and questionable increased leftsided deep tendon reflexes. At follow-up evaluation two weeks after discharge, he reported a mild, dull intermittent pain in the left temple. Neurologic examination revealed no abnormalities.

Migraine Following Athletic Trauma

In 1972 Matthews[154] described a form of migraine that is elicited by blows to the head in soccer or football and in boxing. Two minutes after being accidentally hit by a ball, a soccer player developed tunnel vision lasting for an hour accompanied by tingling in one hand and face, followed by severe headache and vomiting. Almost identical episodes had occurred during the preceding six years. Another player, aged 22, after heading the ball experienced episodes of blurred vision, with the peripheral field "like being under water." After about 30 minutes, this would be followed by severe headache.

Matthews refers to a report by Whitty on another patient who had migraine induced by boxing and to a report by Graham on "youngsters with classical migraine who develop a characteristic attack when hit on the head in a football match." Matthews believes that unexpected blows to the head may cause traction on the arteries at the base of the brain followed by arterial spasm. Unexpected blows to the side of the head are more likely to cause arterial distortion than anticipated and controlled impact, e.g., during skilled heading in soccer.

CATAPLECTIC LOSS OF MUSCLE TONE

Sudden unheralded attacks of loss of muscle tone triggered by emotional excitement occur during athletic competitions. A quarter mile runner was leading by four yards and looked like a sure winner when, 10 yards before the tape, his legs gave in and he fell to the ground unable to move. He was conscious throughout, got up without help after a few seconds. The same kind of col-

lapse took place during the track meet of Britain versus Germany in 1935 when the 400 m finalist, A.K. Brown, inexplicably lost control over his leg muscles and stumbled, unable to finish the race. There too was no impairment of consciousness. The syndrome is indistinguishable from cataplectic collapses of patients with narcolepsy. (E. Jokl[155])

The most usual type of attack of loss of tone and power is that in which on the heels of emotional excitement an atonic powerless state of somatic muscles develops. Knees are relaxed and the patient sinks to the ground though in possession of his senses. One of my patients remarked: 'If I try during a soccer game to shoot the ball at the goal and I see the fellows watching me, the use goes out of my right leg. I simply can't do it.' Another reported that he 'felt all power leave his arm at the moment of serving in a game of tennis. (K. Wilson[156])

The cataplectic attack is a peculiar reaction to happy or sad emotions consisting of sudden loss of tone of the muscles and inability to move voluntarily. In one case a man who was fishing from a boat suffered a typical seizure when on feeling a pull on the line he lost control and fell over-board. In another instance, a wrestler went limp during a match. In still another, a hunter became powerless when he was about to pull the trigger of his gun. A tennis player fell to the ground when he intended to hit a smash ball. (J. Wilder[157])

Beamon's Collapse[158]

At the 1968 Olympic Games in Mexico City, Bob Beamon won the Gold Medal in the long jump with a leap of 8.90 m (29 ft, 2$\frac{1}{2}$ in). His performance which established a new world record ranks as one of the most remarkable athletic feats of all time. It represents an event of special interest to physiology because it is the first athletic performance that stands close to the terminal point of the growth curve of a world record.

I was present at Beamon's jump which electrified everyone who witnessed it. I sensed that something unprecedented had happened. During the ensuing minutes a cluster of officials assembled around the jumping pit, waiting for the arrival of a tape measure — the specially installed semi-automatic Cantabrian recording unit proved to be too short. When Beamon was told that he had jumped 29 ft, 2$\frac{1}{2}$ in, he dropped to the ground as if struck by lightning. He did not lose consciousness, awareness remained unaffected throughout. A similar attack occurred to the winner in the ski jumping competition at the Olympic Winter Games in Grenoble on February 18, 1968,

Vladimir Belusov. Following the announcement of his victory, Belusov collapsed and was unable to rise to his feet; he remained conscious throughout the syncope.

"Powerless attacks" are typical — even though not frequently observed — collapse syndrome of athletes, first described in 1936.[155] Textbooks of clinical neurology refer to them as "cataplectic loss of muscle tone" that occurs as an unusual physical manifestation of emotional excitement in normal subjects. Cataplectic seizures are an ubiquitous accompaniment of narcolepsy.

Beamon's cataplectic collapse represents a psychosomatic model: his syncope was triggered verbally. The announcement that he had jumped 8.90 m in no way seemed to affect him. Like most Americans, he was unable to comprehend metric data. It was only when he was told that he jumped 29 ft, 2¹/₂ that he reacted. Similar collapses are fairly well known. Some have been described in a dramatic setting, e.g., in Gerhart Hauptmann's "Before Sunset."

Every athlete who competed in sprints and other contests of short duration at Mexico City benefitted from the altitude environment: the six finalists in the long jump surpassed the eight meter mark, a feat that was not reached before in Tokyo in 1964 nor at Munich in 1972.

Beamon's jump surpassed the previous world record by an unprecedented margin. Improvement of world records generally upgrades the preceding best performance by a predictable amount. I have referred to Beamon's jump as a "mutation phenomenon" because it did not seem to follow nor could it have been predicted from the chronological sequence of the preceding growth of world records.

That during the years after 1968 the world's best athletes would improve long jumping record standards I took for granted — all world records of track and field records were (and still are) in their developmental stage, even though some of them are far advanced. The record growth curve of the world's best long jumpers "after Beamon" has entered its asymptotic deflection phase: it has reached — or is about to reach — its terminal horizontality.

Carl Lewis, currently the most outstanding American track and field athlete, is about to equal Beamon's 1968 record; he may surpass it, but if so the advancement will occur by a small margin. Because of the unprecedented superiority to the performances of the world's best long jumper of Beamon's feat, I have referred to his as a "genius" achievement — the term "genius" being traditionally applied to human attainments that stand far above the endeavours of their peers. The appearance of geniuses is a rare event. It is all the more remarkable that a decade after Beamon's record jump another athlete has appeared on the competitive scene to whom the same attribute applies: Carl Lewis. The magnitude of his superiority to the best long jumpers of his time is even greater than Beamon's was in the late sixties. In 1983 the second best long jump was more than half a meter less than Lewis' best.

Beamon's syncope did not threaten his life. He was healthy, his coronary arteries and his myocardium were unimpaired. A like collapse in a patient with ischemic heart disease may have different consequences. On October 19, 1973, a 64-year-old golfer in Fullerton, California shot a hole-in-one whereupon he collapsed and died "of an apparent heart attack." Companions said that "the elated sportsman fell to the ground after he got his ace shot."

A Factor Analysis

Beamon's 8.90 meter jump — his best preceding leap had been about half a meter less — was facilitated through a heightened sensitivity level of the "Ascending Reticular Activating System" of the brain (ARAS); and the general lowering of reflex thresholds at altitude. Both represent modalities of "heterostatic" deployment of a special kind. Their simultaneous occurrence engendered a stigmatized situation. ARAS mediates awareness through a cerebral mechanism described in 1949 by Moruzzi and Magoun.[159] These investigators demonstrated the dependence of awareness upon the functional integrity of the "reticular formation" of the brainstem. Electrical stimulation of ARAS causes changes of the electroencephalogram indistinguishable from those that occur during awakening. ARAS also controls the tonic innervation of the anti-gravity muscles of the extremities; both functional resources are activated while we wake up; both are inactivated while we fall asleep. Deliberate sensitization of awareness characterizes certain athletic situations. Contestants who prepare themselves for a jump "sensitize" themselves through a self-designed ritual of concentration, often accompanied by seemingly purposeless gestures. They thus try to establish a basis for the ensuing "disciplined disinhibition" of their motor system.

The second modality of facilitation of the jump to which reference has been made before is the lowering at altitude of reflex thresholds first described in 1933.[160] At that time reflexes were tested on a group of students at Muottas Muraigl, a 2,500 meter summit above Pontresina in Engadin, Switzerland. Control measurements were taken at sea level and at Davos (elevation, 1,600 meters). Reduced atmospheric and partial oxygen pressure cause a shortening of the duration of all tendon reflexes. The phenomenon can be demonstrated with the help of a recording device that employs a beam of light falling on a photoelectric cell.[161] The extent to which these two neural mechanisms combined to produce the "stigmatized" state in which Beamon jumped 8.90 meters was demonstrated by the cataplectic seizure after the record performance.

PRIMARY LOSS OF CONSCIOUSNESS

Sudden primary loss of consciousness, presumably due to the combined effect of hypoxia and acapnia upon the reticular formation in the brainstem, was first described in 1936.[155] Seizures of the kind under reference occur after exhausting competitive performances. They represent mirror images, as it were, of the "arousal reaction" that is mediated through the ascending connections of the reticular formation of the brainstem. In contrast to shock collapse gravitatory displacement of blood does not play a part in the initiation of this syndrome.

A dramatic instance of sudden primary loss of consciousness in Mexico City was Ron Clarke's syncope after the 10,000 meter final in which he finished sixth in 29 minutes, 44.8 seconds, more than two minutes slower than his world record. He was deeply unconscious, looked ashen grey, corneal reflexes could not be elicited. He regained consciousness after a quarter of an hour, was *aphasic* for more than one hour, and unable to recall the last four laps of the race.

A like collapse occurred in the British runner, Maurice Herriott, after the 3,000 meter steeplechase, also at Mexico City.

Primary loss of consciousness after prolonged exhausting athletic performances presents itself often as a dramatic event. The collapse is most likely to occur at the end of exceptionally demanding performances. My previous monograph on "Syncope in Athletes"[13] contains several descriptions of these collapses including that of the Italian runner, Dorando, a few yards before the finishing line at the 1908 Olympic marathon. I have witnessed several like collapses, among them three after the final 1,500 meter event of the Olympic decathlon, six at the "Triathlon" in Hawaii, one after a 200 kilometer bicycle road race, and the two in Mexico City mentioned earlier.

There have so far been no occasions to take EEGs from athletes during primary loss of consciousness. Disturbances of speech and of memory after the seizure represent noteworthy neurological symptoms. In no instance has there been acute cardiac failure. My own hypothesis is that metabolic and thermoregulatory stress can impair the functional integrity of the brainstem reticular formation and its control of consciousness; of the upright posture; and also of its connections with the temporal and parietal lobes of the cerebral cortex.

A reference must still be made to states of impaired awareness in athletes during performances such as marathon running, bicycle races, channel swimming, and mountaineering. These states represent a neurological category of their own because although it is true that the maintenance of both consciousness and of the upright posture are mediated through the brainstem, the observations under reference suggest the connection between the two can be severed: during cataplectic collapses consciousness is maintained while tone of muscles is lost; while all states of unconsciousness muscle tone is lost during the absence of awareness. Spells of amnesia such as those observed in athletes do not necessarily render continuation of running or swimming or other activities impossible. That the athletes' awareness had been affected during their performances is often discovered only after their completion.

Gowers wrote in 1907[162] that "epilepsy and cardiovascular syncope must have a common meeting place in the brain," and that "the line between fits and faints cannot be sharply drawn." It is all the more important to take cognizance of the different combinations of impairment of awareness and muscle tone that offer themselves for observation with athletes under stress.

Loss of Consciousness and Death Due to Cerebral Hemorrhage

After running 10 miles a 14-year-old schoolboy collapses because of right-sided weakness. On arrival at hospital he was dysphasic with right hemiplega. CT showed low-density areas in the territory of the left middle cerebral artery suggesting early infarction. Carotid angiography after 48 hours revealed delayed filling and incomplete opacification of ascending branches of the left middle cerebral artery. Patient was discharged on 12th day. (J. Phillips, B. Horner, T. Doorly, et al.[163])

Chester and Conlong[164] reported two deaths from acute cerebral accidents. Both experienced headache while running followed by a left hemiplegia and by unilateral homonymous hemianopsia and weakness on the left side of the body. No postmortem data were available.

The most likely cause of the deaths is rupture of a congenital intracerebral aneurysm.[165] Chester and Conlon also described the case of a 34-year-old jugger who developed a hemorrhage in the thalamic region of the right cerebral hemisphere, and two cases in which blood stained cerebrospinal fluid was found after athletic effort. Spontaneous intracranial hemorrhages in runners have been seen by Kelly and Roussak.[166]

None of the above events represent physiological sequelae of exercise.

PHYSIOLOGICAL ASPECTS OF THE EDINBURGH COMMONWEALTH GAMES (A.L. MUIR, ET AL.[167])

After any long-distance event, and sometimes after middle-distance events, competitors may need assistance from the track and a period of up to an hour in a nearby recovery room before they are fit to return to their quarters. After the marathon six athletes were taken to the medical treatment center in the stadium — one stated simply that he felt very tired, one reported abdominal pain and diarrhea, the others complained of nausea and sickness. These athletes had cold skins but their blood pressures and heart rates were normal. All such patients require careful medical examination, but rest and hot tea are usually all the treatment needed.

More serious collapses may be due to hyperpyrexia, hypoglycemia, and dehydration. Only two cases of collapses required medical treatment during the games.

The first patient was a Tamil from Singapore who came in 16th in the 20 mile (32 km) walk; he was in front of several competitors, and in a national event his performance would be rated as good. On completing the walk, he reported to his trainer and put on his tracksuit. After an unknown interval of time he was found unconscious in the tunnel leading off the track. His skin was cold, pulse rate 72 per minute, blood pressure 80/60 mm Hg, rectal temperature 38°C. He was treated at once with 1 liter of 5% dextrose and 1 liter of Ringer lactate intravenously, made warm and admitted to the Royal Infirmary. On recovery he gave a history of sore throat and feeling unwell for the previous 2 days; his fauces were infected and he had a slight pyrexia. Biochemical investigations on blood taken at the time of collapse revealed a normal blood sugar but plasma-urea was high (71 mg per 100 ml). No other abnormality was found.

This episode illustrated the possible danger of taking part in athletics when suffering from even a minor infection, and the importance of having facilities for resuscitation beside the track. The mechanism responsible for this collapse remains subject to speculation. Perhaps the fall in cardiac output after the cessation of walking was not accompanied by adequate inhibition of the previously high muscle blood-flow.

The other athlete requiring medical attention was a marathon runner who continued to vomit after the race, and since his condition caused some concern, he was admitted to the hospital. This athlete came in eleventh and established his country's national record. On admission, his blood pressure was 110/80 mm Hg, skin cold and clammy, and rectal temperature 39°C. Apart from some abdominal tenderness there were no abnormal physical signs. He was treated with an antiemetic and settled quickly. His hematocrit reading was 42%. Three hours after the end of the race and without intravenous fluid replacement he passed urine with an osmolality of 450 mosmole per liter.

"Functional Hemiplegia"

A reference must be made to the fact that the left cerebral hemisphere is distinctly more susceptible to physical exhaustion that the right which has no access to awareness and to speech. The collapse syndrome presented at Los Angeles in 1984 by the Swiss woman marathon runner Andersen-Schiess exemplified the pathophysiological result: ataxia, unconsciousness, functional hemiplegia (upper body bent towards the left), followed by complete recovery within hours after the race. I have referred to the syndrome as functional hemiplegia.

Chapter IV

THE IMMUNOLOGICAL STATUS
OF ATHLETES

During the influenza epidemic of 1918-19 among the men serving with the United States Overseas Expeditionary Force a large number of well-trained athletes became afflicted. Many of them died. (H. Zinsser[168])

MONTE CARLO. Miss Nancy Riach, the 20 year old Scottish swimming champion, who was ill with infantile paralysis, died here early today. She was taken ill while competing in the European swimming championships last week. Miss Riach had been regarded as one of Britain's main hopes for next year's Olympic Games at Wembley. She held the British (native) records over 100 yards, 150 yards, 300 yards and 500 yards.

Miss Riach, who competed in the heats of the 100 meters free style against the advice of her doctor failed to qualify for the final. Immediately after this race the doctor ordered her to bed. She had been suffering for several days from what was thought to be a stomach ailment, and had been given an injection before she entered the water Friday. (The Times[169])

Rosie Mittermeir, threefold Olympic Medal winner at Innsbruck in 1972 came down with a severe bout of influenza the day after her last competitions.

After establishing in 1982 one of the most remarkable track running world records of the past decade (5000 meters in 13:00.42), Dave Moorcraft became afflicted with viral hepatitis.

During my ascent of Kangchenzoenge (8585 meters) in Nepal in 1980 my life was threatened by an amoebic infection causing pneumonia and hepatitis. (Reinhold Messner)

A DISCUSSION of the immunological status of athletes in cardiology is justified for several reasons, among them that of the ubiquitous involvement of the heart in infectious diseases;[170] and because of the fact — not generally known among clinicians — that athletes are particularly susceptible to infection.[171]

Serological Studies

Early in the century a number of humoral agents were identified in the human blood distinguished by their ability to mediate a variety of serological reactions. Chief among them are agglutinins, antigens, bacteriolysins, complements, opsonins, phagocytes, precipitins, and tropines; often referred to as "immune bodies." Until the early thirties it was believed that these agents determine the individual's immunological status, an assumption that was proved erroneous through serological studies with athletes.[172] Quantitative assessment of the "immune bodies" failed to show a correlation between their concentration in the blood and health and performance status of trained sportsmen and of untrained controls. The scatter distribution of measurements obtained in analyses of blood of world champion skiers and ice hockey players was the same as that of measurements obtained from analyses of blood of untrained controls and of a group of patients of a tuberculosis sanatorium. Evidently the agents under study are not designed to prevent or cure infectious diseases. R.L. Green, et al.[173] studied immunoglobulins (IgG, IgA, IgM), leukocyte phagocytosis in twenty marathon runners. C_3, C_4, properdin factor B, T, and B cells and phytohemagglutinin and pokeweed mitogen stimulation of lymphocytes were determined. Complete blood counts, including platelets, were obtained. All results were within normal limits. None of the findings correlated with the incidence of infectious diseases among the athletes. The authors concluded that "long distance running has no effect on immune function."

During the 1968 Olympic Games in Mexico City, an epidemic of enteritis incapacitated more than a quarter of the athletes. The illness was more severe in participants than among visitors. An epidemic of influenza occurred at the Olympic Winter Games in Innsbruck in 1972, severely affecting many of the world's best skiers and ice hockey players.

The effectiveness — within the strict limits of their specific functional characteristics — of all serological components of the blood is temporarily increased by exercise.[174] The increases are due to the mobilization during exercise of the autonomic nervous system, a phenomenon referred to by Walter Cannon as the Emergency Function of the Adreno-Sympathetic System.[175]

Important facets of this interplay of physiological responses and pathological processes have been elucidated in studies of the deleterious effect of strenuous physical activity upon viral diseases, especially poliomyelitis and hepatitis, also of influenza, the most common cause of incapacitation of athletes through infections, often accompanied by myocarditis.

Poliomyelitis

In 1937 De Rudder and Petersen[176] observed an acute outbreak of infantile paralysis in a boarding school in a small town. Of 107 boarders of a hostel who proceeded by bicycle or on foot to a neighboring town to compete in an athletic meeting lasting several days, twenty-one fell victims to infantile paralysis. All of them had undergone severe physical strain immediately prior to the onset of the illness. A group morbidity of more than twenty percent is a rate previously unheard of in connection with infantile paralysis. Even in the most severe epidemics so far known the highest incidence observed in a town was 0.5 percent, including abortive cases without paralysis. Apart from the cases affecting boys living in one hostel, not a single instance of poliomyelitis was reported in the neighborhood, although there were in the same town a primary school as well as another boys' hostel, not to speak of the rest of the population.

In 1945 Levinson, et al.[177] summarized reports available at the time in the literature supporting the impression that chilling and physical activity towards the end of the incubation period of poliomyelitis sharply increases the incidence of quadriplegia and death. They subjected monkeys to exhausting exercise (swimming) during the incubation period of experimental poliomyelitis. A higher incidence or more severe paralysis occurred in the exercised animals than in controls.

In 1947 Ritchie Russell[178] presented a paper entitled, "Poliomyelitis: The Pre-paralytic Stage, and the Effect of Physical Activity on the Severity of Paralysis," based upon an analysis of observations made during the last major polio epidemic in Great Britain. Russell referred to the fact that a history of great physical exertion preceding

the onset of severe paralysis had evoked comment in cases of poliomyelitis but that no attempt had been made to investigate this aspect of the problem statistically. The paper contains an analysis of
meningitic symptoms, pain in the head, spine, trunk or thighs, into
"paralysis gradings," namely, patients with full recovery and patients
with "residual impairment of the disease." It concluded that "physical
activity in the pre-paralytic stage of the disease greatly reduces the
resistance of the spinal cord cells to the virus and should therefore be
avoided at all costs."

Hargreaves[179] concurred with the conclusion drawn by Russell in
1947 that "severe physical activity during the pre-paralytic stage of
poliomyelitis is associated with grave prognosis. Severe mental
strain such as driving a car over long distances, appears to be
equally disastrous, whereas paralysis tends to be mild in cases confined to bed during the pre-paralytic stage."

In 1949 Russell[180] presented a follow-up study entitled, "Paralytic
Poliomyelitis: The Early Symptoms and the Effect of Physical Activity on the Course of the Disease," based upon questioning of one
hundred convalescents of poliomyelitis, fifty-nine males and forty-
one females. Three stages of the disease were analyzed separately:
the prodromal, the pre-paralytic, and the paralytic.

Russell points out that the pre-paralytic stage begins abruptly,
gets worse for two, three or more days, and culminates in paralysis.
Subjectively, the patient may feel better when paralysis develops
with the result "that often those who continue physical activity after
the symptoms begin either are relatively insensitive to pain or have
more than the average courage, or incentive to continue to work or
play in spite of illness. There is certainly no doubt that many of
those most severely crippled have remarkable strength of character
and great powers of endurance. It has been said that the disease
picks the best child of the family."

The statistical evidence indicated once more that complete physical rest from the onset of symptoms will seldom fail to prevent serious paralysis while strenuous or even moderate physical activity is
highly dangerous.

Complete physical rest in bed from the onset of the pre-paralytic
stage greatly reduces the danger of severe paralysis. Severe physical
activity at this stage is almost suicidal, while the continuance of even

average physical activity is dangerous. The highly dangerous belief that malaise and other vague symptoms should be "worked off" by exercise requires correction.

In 1951 E.C. Parker Williams[181] reported on the case of a second attack of poliomyelitis precipitated by violent exercise.

A recently qualified physician of "distinctive athletic ability" had suffered the first mild attack of poliomyelitis in September 1947. There was moderate neck rigidity and a positive Kernig sing, some weakness of the left triceps and left extensor carpi radialis and of the left foot. The patient made an excellent recovery. On January 19, 1950, he engaged in a violent game of squash after which he developed a severe headache and later vomited. Marked meningitic symptoms set in: there was tenderness over occipital and trapezius muscles, and his temperature rose to 100.4. On January 22 the condition worsened rapidly and respiratory embarrassment necessitated placement in a Both respirator. The following day he died of cardiac and respiratory failure.

It is possible that had he remained quietly in bed during the remission, the illness would have terminated and aborted an attack of poliomyelitis without paralysis.

In 1973 Weinstein[182] described an epidemic of poliomyelitis in a private school in Greenwich, Connecticut which occurred between September 29 and October 17, 1972. Because of religious convictions none of the students, faculty, and other members of the staff of the school had received any kind of immunization against poliomyelitis. Eleven children were afflicted: two girls, 7 and 12 years, and nine boys of between 12 and 18 years of age, all of them members of the school's football team. Without exception the boys developed paralysis of extemities. Weinstein writes that the 100% incidence of paralysis in the boys was probably related to their participation in strenuous sports.

Hepatitis

Hepatitis has many epidemiological similarities to poliomyelitis. Both are enteric infections associated with viremia, with localization in one system, liver or central nervous system. The effect of exercise during the early stages of the disease represents another similarity. Krikler and Zilberg[188] presented evidence showing that exercise facilitates the development of the fulminant manifestations of hepatitis and that vigorous physical activity may be responsible for a fatal outcome. In less severe cases, strenuous exercise is not likely to be a feature.

The authors presented the histories of five patients who had engaged in strenuous exercise when the first symptoms of the illness appeared. Two had been keen athletes. One played cricket all day and danced at night, despite mild malaise. The next morning he was feverish and jaundiced, restless, vomited, became stuporous and died the following day. A girl who took part in school sports fell ill three days after with nausea and vomiting, followed by jaundice, delirium and coma. Another patient went yachting despite malaise, came into a gale which required extremely strenuous effort. The following day he felt nauseated and became jaundiced; death set in two days later. A fourth patient played rugby immediately prior to the onset of the terminal illness. A fifth was a young woman who had begun spring cleaning the day she fell ill. She did not stop working despite the onset of jaundice. She died in the hospital.[183]

In 1972 Morse[184] observed a hepatitis outbreak involving most members of a college football team. The pathogenic virus had been transmitted by polluted drinking water.

Aseptic Meningitis with Echovirus-16 Infection

One must consider that the severity of enteroviral disease may be enhanced in groups who engage in strenuous physical exertions. (Baron, et al.)[185]

Baron, et al.[185] observed an outbreak of aseptic meningitis associated with echovirus-16 infection among members of a high school football team. In an epidemiological analysis all fifty-eight football players from a North Carolina high school were compared with a group consisting of the same number of non-team pupils. The enteroviral illness of team members was distinctly more severe than that of the control group, showing that membership on the football team was associated with an increased incidence of an aseptic meningitis-like syndrome that resulted in the hospitalization of seven players. Enterovirus was recovered from players with neurological syndromes, from those principally with respiratory symptoms, as well as from asymptomatic players. Pupils not on the team experienced symptoms of an aseptic meningitis-like syndrome that were milder, but similar to those experienced by team members. None of them required hospitalization. Excessive illness and aseptic meningitis had clustered among members of the football team.

Clinical and laboratory observations have suggested that physical exertion during incubation and prodromal periods may result in more severe enteroviral illness of many kinds. Mice forced to exercise after they were infected with coxsackievirus A9 demonstrated increased virus proliferation in myocardial tissue, and mice exercised after infection with coxsackievirus B3 had increased virus proliferation in the myocardium and experienced greater mortality.

All viral diseases have in common that they interfere with physical activities. Athletes thus afflicted invariably note that they are ill and out of form. In cases of infectious mononucleosis, a frequent cause of incapacitation, restriction of activities should be maintained until the febrile phase is over and until any splenic enlargement or tenderness has been absent for at least a week. A major concern is possible rupture of the spleen from abdominal trauma.[186]

Cold, Influenza and Respiratory Diseases

During the eighth week of the "Kentucky Fitness Experiment" in 1959 on the effect of daily physical training on the physical and mental status of adolescent boys and girls, a severe influenza epidemic struck the community. Between February 26, 1959, and March 16, 1959, almost half of the class population were absent from school. The normal absentee ratio of 2-6% rose to an unprecedented 42-46%.

The impact of the epidemic was the same upon the trained children and the controls. The fact that, as a result of the preceding period of training, the level of fitness of the experimental groups had significantly improved, did not reveal itself as being of protective value. Number of days of absenteeisms were the same in the experimental group and in the controls.[187]

Tuberculosis

The incidence of pulmonary tuberculosis has been sharply reduced during recent years. However, it is appropriate to point out tuberculosis was a fairly frequent occurrence among athletes until a few decades ago.

In 1942 Dormer, et al.[188] who examined the files of the King George V Hospital in Durban, found several cases of advanced pulmonary tuberculosis in young athletes. They pointed out that the disease inevitably causes deterioration of physical efficiency.

> A 24-year-old pilot who had been a first class tennis player was admitted to the hospital because of lancinating pains in the left side of the chest. X-ray examination of the chest revealed massive disease of the left lung, sputum contained numerous tubercle bacilli.

> A 37-year-old man who had been accustomed to vigorous exercise for several years noted a marked decrease in his athletic efficiency, got breathless when he ran, and could no longer swim his usual daily 600 yards. X-ray examination revealed a large cavity at the apex of the left lung.

> Other cases pertained to a 36-year-old stoker on a tug; a 25-year-old sailor; a 29-year-old nurse; and an 18-year-old high school tennis player who presented similar histories. The last named patient consulted a physician because of loss of weight, and short windedness; her menses which had been regular did not appear during recent months.

Vaccinia

An editorial note in *The Lancet*, November 20, 1948[189] commented on a case of vaccinia after boxing. A young Norwegian soldier had been vaccinated against smallpox in childhood and came to England on September 8, 1948, as a member of an Army athletic team. On the 20th he noticed a rash on his face, but did not feel ill; before returning to Norway he indulged in much sight-seeing, visiting among other places the House of Commons. On his return to Norway the rash had developed into a pustular eruption and he was admitted to the Ullevaal Hospital on September 25. The pustulas eruption on his head, neck, and right upper arm must it was thought be due to one of two things — vaccinia or variola. Material from the eruption was sent by air to London for laboratory tests which revealed the infection to be vaccinial. Reporting the case to the Norwegian Medical Society on November 3, Dr. Per Hanssen suggested that there may have been vaccinia pus on the boxing gloves of one or other of the three men with whom the patient boxed in London a few days before the first appearance of the rash. The length of the interval between the boxing and the appearance of the rash, and its limitation to just those parts of the body which are most exposed to abrasions during boxing, supported this explanation.

Dermatological Disorders

A survey of dermatological disorders in athletes presented by Ruch[190] contained descriptions of contact dermatitis caused by agents such as tincture of benzoin, mercury compounds, liniments, dyes, leather, rubber, adhesive tape, plastic materials, lime and chalk; verrucae which disable by reason of both location and size; molluscum contagiosum, viral lesions caused by contaminated towels which may appear most commonly on the trunk; foot infections, both bacterial and fungous; pyoderma and epidemic cutaneous herpes simplex (herpes Gladiatorum),[191,192] occurring often in wrestlers, Vincent's disease, producing acute edematous and vesicular inflammation of the mouth, caused by the fusiform bacillus and Spirillum Vincentii; moniliasis, a moderately severe dermatitis usually in the groins and axillae with Candida albicans acting as infecting microorganism; and miliaria rubra, seen most frequently in basketball players and runners who sweat a great deal.

An epidemic of pyoderma in football players caused by nephritogenic streptococci was studied by Glezen, et al.[193] The organism produced lesions consisting of septic abrasions and infected lacerations. The causative bacterium was an M-type 2 streptococcus with antigenic characteristics similar to those associated with acute glomerulonephritis following pyoderma in children.

Participants in the Swedish Cross Country Running Championship in Gothenburg were examined with a view to obtaining information on the incidence of pyoderma caused by the Staphylococcus pyogenes aureus and the beta-hemolytic streptococcus. Fifty-two runners, among them several of the best, reported that at some time or another they had suffered from the dermatological complaint under study. A subsequent inquiry revealed that 260 out of 950 Swedish cross country runners had been afflicted with pyoderma. The spread of the disease is confined to the autumn and coincides with the peak of morbidity of impetigo contagiosa. The reason is that cross country running starts after conclusion of the summer season. (Sieler[194])

Herpes Simplex Virus Type 1

William B. White, et al. emphasized that skin infections, both bacterial and viral, are endemic in contact sports such as wrestling and rugby football. They described four cases of extensive cutaneous herpes simplex virus in players on a rugby team. All had a prodrome of fever, malaise, and anorexia with a weight loss of 3.6 to 9.0 kg. Two players experienced ocular lesions associated with cutaneous vesicular lesions of the face. A third player, who had herpetic lesions on his lower extemity, experienced paresthesias, weakness, and intermittent urinary retention. All infected players on the team were forwards or members of the "scrum," which suggests a field-acquired infection analogous to the herpetic infections seen in wrestlers (herpes Gladiatorum). The authors concluded that considering the serious sequelae of recurrent herpes simplex keratitis, the traumatic skin lesions in rugby football players should be cultured for herpes virus, and infected individuals should be restricted from playing until crusted lesions have disappeared.[195]

SCABIES AND IMPETIGO

Several years ago a comprehensive study of the "Physical Health and Social Status of 'Good' and 'Bad' Pupils" was conducted.[196] It yielded information on the determining influence of socioeconomic environment upon growth and development of young children, with the incidence of scabies and impetigo representing a "label" identifying neglected children from poor urban homes.

One hundred and twenty-seven children 6-7 years of age were divided into three groups in accordance with their scholastic status at school. All of them came from the same poor urban district of Johannesburg and represented a sociologically homogeneous group. Each child's class performances were marked after the pupils had been at school for six months, and a second time half a year later. The dullest group scored significantly lower than the middle and the brightest groups. There were statistically significant differences in respect of bodily growth, rates of absenteeism, physical efficiency, home conditions, and economic status: the brightest group ranked well above the others throughout. Also, the bright pupils were significantly superior in respect of the incidence of normal skins as against cutaneous manifestations of malnutrition, of scabies and impetigo, of conjunctivitis and eye discharges, and of inflammation of the pharynx.

Standard tests of physical efficiency (running over 100 and 600 yards and putting the 12 pound shot) revealed no signficant differences between the three groups at the beginning of the first school terms. At the end of the year, however, the bright pupils were leading. They had made the greatest performance progress. This result corroborated a previous finding by Milne, et al.[197] that no physiological correlation exists between basic intellectual and physical efficiency of school children. However the evidence obtained in the study under review suggested a better physical educability of the good pupils.

Race Horses

In the context of the discussion of the immunological status of athletes, a reference is appropriate to the great susceptibility of the world's best race horses. Like human athletes, they too are not in possession of enhanced powers of resistance against pathogenic microorganisms.

Contagious Equine Metritis (CEM)

Two outbreaks of highly contagious equine metritis among racing horses of world class occurred in 1977 and 1978, the one on stud farms in the Newmarket area in England[198] and the other in the Bluegrass country of Kentucky[199]. The CEM organism is spread not only in sexual contact but also by handlers and through contact with exposed material. Stallions are not affected by it, they only act as carriers. In mares it causes infection of the endometrium of the uterus which often results in failure to conceive or to come to term.

Equine Viral Arteritis

During the end of May 1984, an epidemic of viral disease called "equine viral arteritis" occurred among thoroughbred horses in Kentucky. It affected a large number of racing horses in the Bluegrass region and led to a ban on thoroughbreds scheduled to be imported to Europe from the United States. The disease causes abortion and severely incapacitates thoroughbred horses for several months.

Amebic Meningo-Encephalitis

Cerva, et al.[200] investigated an epidemic of amoebic meningo-encephalitis due to infestation of an indoor pool with amoebae which resembled the organism described as Hartmannella or Naegleria. The epidemic had caused sixteen deaths. The pathogenic amoebae were seen at autopsy:

> In the brain tissue of all victims amebas were found which corresponded morphologically to amebas of the limax group. In all cases the meninges were massively infiltrated, especially by polynuclear leukocytes. Damage to the walls of blood vessels was relatively rare. There were a rather large number of globular formations of amorphous masses corresponding in size and staining character to the cytoplasm of amebas in the leukocytic infiltrate. More rarely, in these masses the typical nuclei of amebas or whole amebas in various degrees of destruction were visible in vacuoles of large mononuclear phagocytes. Characteristic is the penetration of amebas into the cerebral cortex through perivascular spaces even along the finest capillaries. In the vicinity of the affected vessels there was a leukocytic infiltration, mostly of neutrophils, following rather closely behind the amebic invasion. The cerebral cortex is damaged to a considerable depth, the basal parts being affected especially markedly. Regularly the cerebellum was heavily infiltrated by amebas, which definitely preferred and destroyed the ganglial and granular layer. Also, the spinal cord surface was invariably affected by infiltration of amebas. The spinal cord itself usually was little affected.

> The localization and number of amebas, the extent of lesions of the CNS tissues, and the cellular reaction evoked by the presence of parasites are evidence of the decisive role played by the amebas in the development of the symptoms of the disease and the death of the patients.

No like epidemic outbreak of the disease had previously been observed even though amebic meningo-encephalitis in swimmers was known to occur sporadically. Sixteen solitary instances were recorded between 1937 and 1971 in persons who had swum in the fresh water lakes around Richmond, Virginia. A case study of amebic meningo-encephalitis was undertaken by Ruma, et al.[201] C.G. Butt[202] described three cases of primary amebic meningo-encephalitis in young men resulting from prolonged swimming in tepid lake-water. He stressed the common etiologic pattern of intranasal inoculation.

Two cases of primary amebic meningo-encephalitis were reported by the U.S. Center for Disease Control in Atlanta. The one referred to a 14-year-old boy who had been swimming in a fresh water lake in Florida for the past three weeks. He complained of progressive severe frontal and bitemporal headache, developed fever and malaise and was admitted to a hospital with nuchal rigidity and lethargy. Examination of the CSF revealed motile amebae. The patient deteriorated rapidly, became disoriented, agitated and comatose. He developed cerebral edema and herniation; he died three days after admission.

The other case was that of a nine-year-old girl who had bathed in a hot spring near San Bernardino in California. She was hospitalized with a three-day history of headache, nausea, vomiting, lethargy, and stupor. Examination of CSF revealed motile amebae. She recovered completely within a month having been treated with intravenous and intrathecal amphotericin B, miconazole — effective in vitro against Naegleria — and oral rifampin.[203]

Shigellosis

Another communicative disease that can be acquired through swimming is Shigella gastroenteritis. In 1974, 31 of 45 cases of *Shigella sonnei* infection in Dubuque, Iowa were traced to swimming in the Mississippi River (Rosenberg, et al.[204]). There was a significant correlation between swimming and illness shown by comparison with a control group. The affected subjects had been swimming in water where the fecal coliform count was 17,500 organisma per 100 ml; the federal upper limit for swimming water is 200 per 100 ml.

Sarcoidosis

At autopsy of a 45-year-old marathon runner who had completed several long distance races prior to his fatal collapse active sarcoidosis was found diffusely present throughout lungs and plurae, in the spleen, lymph nodes, liver and bone. The heart was enlarged (510 grams) with symmetrical left ventricular hypertrophy. The two major branches of the left coronary artery were occluded by atheroma without thrombosis. There was subendocardial fibrosis. (Parsons, et al.[205])

Other Parasitic Infections

Other parasitic infections have been noted in athletes. At the post mortem examination of a 12-year-old girl who died unexpectedly after colliding with another player on the basketball court, a freshly torn cyst in the liver was found. Histological examination showed scolices and hooklets in the wall of the cyst. (See also reference 206.)

A case of successful surgical treatment of a cardiac echinococcal cyst was recorded. The diagnosis was made by two-dimensional echocardiography in a 35-year-old man who "denied shortness of breath, cough, syncope, recurrent fever, skin rash, or abdominal symptoms." The encapsulated cyst and the interior pulmonary valve cup to which it was attached were excised. Several electrocardiograms after surgery demonstrated an incomplete right bundle branch block. The patient returned home and did well during a one year follow-up period.[207]

The problem of "swimmer's itch" (cutaneous schistosomiasis) was discussed. Schistosome dermatitis frequently occurs in people who swim in the new Aswan Dam in Egypt.

In a highly successful athlete, Evans[208] discovered massive infestation of the entire musculature with cysticercosis. Hundreds of cysts of varying degrees of calcification were identified in roentgenograms made after the subject had suffered a major epileptic seizure caused by a cyst in the brain.

As mentioned before, susceptibility of athletes to infections is ubiquitous. After his return to London with the British Olympic team from Melbourne in 1956, James Cussen[209] reported that the most irksome troubles he had with the athletes were infections. Nasopharyngeal infections, he wrote, occurred rather frequently if the weather was cold and there was much dust in the air. There were many cases of sore throat, catarrh with closure of the Eustachian tubes and consequent deafness, as well as cough. Skin infections were common. Pimples, boils, carbuncles, impetigo, and tinea of the feet progressing to lymphagitis required attention. As the weather became warmer, gnat bites were frequent and severe inflammatory reactions from them were troublesome. Commenting on his experience in the Olympic Village in Tokyo in 1964, D.F. Hanley[210] mentioned that several athletes from Ghana had chronic malaria and anemia and that their performances were therefore greatly impaired. Olympic participants from other African countries were similarly afflicted. Even among the highly trained U.S. athletes intercurrent infections, particularly of the respiratory, and gastrointestinal systems, and of the skin, ranked as chief medical problems during their stay in Japan. My own experiences at the Mexico City Olympic Games in 1968 corroborated the validity of the above statements.

Because outstanding athletes who compete in international meetings come into physical contact with an exceptional variety of persons and also because of the fact that they travel a great deal, unusual sources of infection must at times be considered.

Maegraith,[211] a professor of tropical medicine in Liverpool, published the case histories of two internationally famous racing cyclists who shortly after their return to England from central Africa fell ill with fever, headache, vomiting, and epigastric discomfort. In both cases, malignant tertian malaria (Plasmodium calciparum) parasites were found in the blood. In the first, treatment was initiated in time and the patient recovered; in the second, the diagnosis could be established only post-mortem. Horniblow[212] who accompanied a joint expedition of the British Army Mountaineering Association and the Pakistan Army of 1959 in northwest Kashmir, reported that several members of the expedition had been afflicted with sore throats, gastroenteritis, septic cutaneous lesions and disturbing fungus infections of the feet. He felt that prospective participants in high mountain expeditions should have their tonsils removed as a prophylactic measure (a procedure no longer recommended), suggested that on their return each climber's stool be examined for bacillary dysentery, amebiasis and ascariasis.

Hanley remarks that among Olympic athletes respiratory and gastro-intestinal infections are the most common infections, with skin infections more prevalent during the summer games. Tinea cruris of a tenacious chronic variety seems to plague cyclists and trackmen, while swimmer's ear (external otitis) is prevalent in both the swimming and water polo teams. Herpes simplex in a wrestler can be a major catastrophe. It disqualifies him from competition.

This contagious virus must not be allowed to contaminate wrestling mats because of the danger of spreading the infection to others through an abraded area of the skin or eye. Dermatophytosis of the feet is present in a chronic semi-controlled state in a large number of athletes, all of whom want to cover it up when what it really needs is soap and water two or three times a day, exposure to the air and sunlight, and frequent changes of clean socks. Scabies is a growing problem: fortunately, it is rarely seen in athletes.

The common cold accounts for 98% of the respiratory tract infections one sees, and therapy for this is a problem. A great many of the usual cold remedies have ephedrine and ephedrine-like compounds or other central nervous system stimulants that are on the "banned list" because of their use as doping agents. They do not contribute anything to improve performance, but the detection of a banned drug in the urine of a competitor will result in disqualification. Several athletes were disqualified at the Games in Munich, and every one of these athletes claimed that medications had been taken because of illness. Most were cases of self-medication, and in a few, the medication had been prescribed by the athlete's personal physician who did not know "the rules of the Games" or thought them unimportant. Tracheitis and bronchitis, and occasionally pneumonia, will account for the other 2% of respiratory tract infections. In a comprehensive analysis of the frequency of respiratory diseases in highly trained athletes in East Germany, Thümmler[213] found that "the most common afflictions are acute infections of the upper respiratory tract."

The gastroenteritis of travelers is an ever-present entity. In one representative sample the attack rate was close to 80%. Prevention is the only answer. Hand-washing after using the toilet, and again before eating, and careful attention to where and what is eaten, with special care as to water and ice sources, and to the containers from which they are consumed will keep the attack rate to a bare minimum. The commonest cause of simple diarrhea is overeating and the consumption of an unusual amount of fresh fruit. The quality and the availability of food at the Olympic Village makes overeating a very real temptation.

Chapter V

THE AGING HEART

No results of macroscopic or microscopic studies of the heart have been reported that are due specifically to aging and that are not also seen in hearts of younger subjects. It is impossible to determine cardiac age with the help of morphological procedures. (A.J. Linzbach)[214,215]

Senior Gymnasts, 1954[216]

A STUDY of the physical and health status of 1,704 participants in the National Festival for Senior Gymnasts in Marburg, Germany (men 40-75; women 30-55) revealed them to be much fitter than untrained young ones.[216] The women gymnasts maintained their physical performance standards unchanged between ages 30 and 45. At the Olympic Games 1960, 1964, 1968, and 1972, a number of grandmothers, all of them strikingly young in appearance, obtained medals. In 1982, forty-seven women aged 55 and older finished the Honolulu marathon. Klaus Jung[217] has reported on observations of over two hundred participants of above 60 years of age in the 100 km (60 miles) run at Biel, Switzerland. Terence Kavanagh[218] has presented a report on middle aged and elderly marathon runners who had undergone prolonged rehabilitative training after myocardial infarction. Evidently, effective responses to training occur not only in healthy subjects but also in subjects afflicted with chronic cardiovascular and other illnesses, irrespective of age. Physical performance standards of large groups of trained athletes and gymnasts of between 40 and 70 years of age are superior to those of untrained subjects half their ages.[219]

Physiology of Aging

In 1938 Robinson[220] observed that the ability of the heart to accelerate with exercise declines with age. A reduction with age of maximal oxygen intake capacity, reflecting a decline of physical endurance, was demonstrated by Hollmann.[221] During the early fifties, a number of physiological parameters were assessed in an unselected sample of men and women of between 30 and 90 years of age, most of them residing in old age homes. Nathan Shock and B.L. Strehler[222] who conducted the study found a consistent decline during the six decades under review of basal metabolic rate, work capacity, cardiac output, vital capacity, maximum breathing volume, nerve conduction velocity, body water content, filtration rate of renal glomeruli, and kidney plasma flow. To reiterate, the subjects under reference in the foregoing were unselected, in contrast to the trained old individuals mentioned earlier.[216]

Age alone gives no information about an individual's mental and physical competence or health. Critical determinants of fitness are freedom from impairing disease, also of course ability and desire to continue to perform during the advancing years. The athletic status of young persons who do not comply with the above prerequisites is inferior to that of old persons who do.

People in the U.S. today live longer due to progress in preventive, diagnostic, therapeutic, and surgical medicine. Further advancements in medicine are likely to increase the current trend. Mohler[223] has pointed out that if cancer were controlled, median age or survival would be 74.8 years; while if heart disease were controlled, median age of survival would be 80.5 years. If vascular lesions, cancer and heart disease were controlled, median age of survival would be 98.8 years.

Earlier concepts of deterioration with age of mental and physical fitness have been based on studies which failed to make the distinction between aging subjects who are free of debilitating illnesses and others who are not.

Aging and Illness

Illnesses represent health problems irrespective of age. It is from studies with older people who are not ill that "the aging process" can be most readily identified, best perhaps in successful old athletes.

The frequency of chronic illnesses in the U.S. for age groups under 45, and 45-64 and over has been assessed. About half of all non-institutionalized persons over 65 have a chronic health condition that limits their activities. Corresponding figures for the age range 45-64 are twenty-four percent; for those younger than 45, seven percent.

Mohler's Report, 1981[223]

The calendar age of 60 is no longer medically justifiable as an upper limit for airline pilots.

Earlier beliefs that powers of physical endurance invariably decline with age must be revised as the participation of large numbers of elderly participants in long distance running events exemplifies. Mohler has raised the issue in another context namely in so far as it relates to existing age limitation for airline pilots.

The calendar age of 60 is no longer medically justifiable as an upper limit for airline pilots. Advances in gerontologic studies, clinical medicine and operational flight proficiency evaluations, now allow individual pilot assessments for health status and performance capability. Individualizing the career duration of pilots by eliminating the present age 60 upper limitation will enhance flight safety and efficiency as the highly qualified, experienced and proficient older, healthy pilots continue their productive careers.

Disabling influences of disease upon "health" for flying personnel are of major interest to cardiology irrespective of age. In the U.S., medical certification for flying is denied if an applicant has an established medical history or clinical diagnosis of any of the following conditions:

1. A personality disorder that is severe enough to have repeatedly manifested itself by overt acts.
2. A psychosis.
3. Alcoholism.
4. Drug dependence.
5. Epilepsy.
6. Disturbance of consciousness without satisfactory medical explanation of the cause.

7. Myocardial infarction.
8. Angina pectoris or other evidence of coronary disease.
9. Diabetes mellitus requiring insulin or other hypoglycemic drug for control.

While the above conditions preclude acceptance for flying duties irrespective of age, the physical and mental status of healthy pilots over 60 is equal or superior to that of younger ones. Older pilots have more experience and are less likely to be involved in accidents.

Robert Kohn[224] has pointed out that in populations over 80, diseases with different etiologies and pathogeneses cause death at a predictable age in that different illnesses such as ischemic heart disease, pneumonia, accidents and cerebrovascular diseases are responsible for death between 85-90 years. (Malignant neoplasms represent an exception in that they cause death over a wide range of ages.) Kohn believes that the enumerated causes of death are merely complications of a fundamental age-related process. The latter, he states "constitutes a 100% fatal disease that every old person has." If people over 80 avoid malignant neoplasms, most will die of ischemic heart disease, cerebrovascular disease, pneumonia, or accidents. While it cannot be predicted of which of these diseases individuals will die, they will die at about the same time. According to Kohn, the organism's ability to adapt itself to environmental demands decreases with age to a level at which life can no longer be maintained, and rather trivial injuries now will cause death. He accepts "senescence" as a common cause of death, due to "profound changes in homeostatic mechanisms."

Physical Activity and Aging

It is in this context that observations of major physical performances of old people such as gymnastics or marathon running deserve special attention. Old athletes seem to be in possession of superior "homeostatic mechanisms," of the kind to which Kohn refers, able to react like younger persons. They live better but not longer. No evidence is available showing that physical activity prolongs life.

During the sixties, Yudkin[225] reported that in England between 1930 and 1960 numbers of radio and TV licenses and of myocardial infarction had increased *pari passu*. The finding did of course not prove that more people were dying because of poor TV programs. Rather, the two trends reflected sequelae of a lifestyle adopted at the time in affluent societies and their careless health habits: smoking, overeating and physical inactivity — all of them identified as coronary risk facts.

"The Aging Brain"

As recently as 1961, Greenfield, et al.[226] wrote in their textbook of Neuropathology that "in old age the brain, in company with all other organs of the body, tends to atrophy."

Is such a statement universally valid? One cannot fail being impressed by the fact that some old people are mentally at their best and that some athletes up to age 80 are fitter than non-athletes half their age. The participants in the gymnastic festival at Marburg of the age group 40-80 certainly did not show signs of cerebral atrophy. Physically active old men and women, of course, represent a sample that is not representative of the older population in its entirety. Nevertheless their existence throws doubt upon the validity of Greenfield, et al.'s description of the brain of old people being marked by widening of cortical sulci; by enlargement of cerebral ventricles; by reduction of cerebral blood circulation; by thickening of the medial layer of arterioles; by formation of argyrophilic plaques and fibrillary tangles; by depigmentation of the substantia nigra; and by progressive reduction of arborisation of dendrites of cortical ganglion cells, alterations said to be particularly noticeable in the hippocampus, whose integrity is a prerequisite for unimpaired memory. If it is true that the response of the brain to aging parallels that of all other organs of the body, one must assume that the brains of old participants in sporting events, in marathon running and long distance swimming, in gymnastics, and weight lifting look better than those who spend their later years in old age homes. No detailed studies have so far been conducted with brains of old athletes and pianists and conductors. At the age of 83, Arturo Toscanini conducted two symphonies in one evening. On his 90th birthday, Arthur Rubinstein played the Second Piano Concerto by Brahms; and at age 92, Lord Philip Noel-Baker delivered a memorable address at the Olympic Congress at Baden-Baden in 1982. The hypothesis is worth considering that "the aging process is amenable to modification with exercise, as other organ systems are amenable to modification with exercise." Diseases of the brain that befall old people — the dementias, Alzheimer's disease and others — are not synonymous with the aging process. As far as the functional status of heart and blood vessels of old men and women is concerned, we know for sure the extent to which it is modifiable through exercise. Undoubtedly old subjects who participate in strenuous athletic events such as long distance running or cycling or swimming or mountaineering represent a population sample of their own. It is likely that most of them are free of severe illnesses and therefore of special interest to students of "the aging heart" and "the aging brain." *

---

* It is appropriate in this context to recall Alzheimer's statement made during the first decade of this century that "arteriosclerotic and senile processes in the brain are unrelated." (Biography of Alois Alzheimer, in W. Haymaker, *Founders of Neurology*. Springfield, Ill., Thomas, 1970.)

Chapter VI

THE HEALTH VALUE OF EXERCISE

Men with angina pectoris naturally try to restrict their physical activity. Thus the least activity class of men is unduly loaded with prime candidates for a heart attack. (Ancel Keyes)[227]

IS exercise able to "cure diseases"? Are joggers immune to myocardial infarction? Are athletes less susceptible to infections than non-athletes? Does the use of physical training in cardiac rehabilitation lead to disappearance of plaques in the coronaries and of scars in the myocardium? What is the explanation of epidemiological findings showing that the cardiac status of physically active persons is superior to that of sedentary populations? What is the role of exercise in geriatric medicine?

Paffenbarger's Epidemiological Studies[228]

Ralph Paffenbarger has conducted two major epidemiological studies both aiming at clarification of the relationship between exercise and cardiac health.

In the first study, about 4,000 longshoremen and dockworkers in San Francisco, 35 to 74 years of age, were examined. Their tasks ranged from supervisory and light machine work to lifting, toting, shoving and stacking. Each of them was given a screening examination when they entered the study in 1951. Five personal characteristics were assessed: cigarette smoking, systolic blood pressure, diagnosed heart disease, weight for height, and glucose metabolism. Job classifications of the longshoremen were documented and energy expenditures required for work tasks calculated. *Low-energy*

91

workers were designated as those who expended fewer than 8,500 kilocalories (Kcal) per week; *high-energy* workers were those who expended 8,500 or more Kcal per week. The men were then followed over a 22-year period to determine rate and risk of fatal heart attack in low-energy and in high-energy workers. Fatal heart attack rates and relative risks were computed and rates of risk for low-energy longshoremen divided by rates of risk for high-energy longshoremen.

The chief result obtained in this study was that men who had expended 8,500 or more Kcal per week had significantly less risk of fatal heart attack than did men whose jobs required less energy output.

The second study was undertaken with Harvard alumni. It covered the period of 1962 to 1972. Experiences and characteristics of alumni who had entered college from 1916 to 1950 were assessed. Information was obtained about cigarette smoking, blood pressure, height and weight, parental death and disease, college varsity athletics, and non-varsity sports play. Data concerning death from heart attacks were available.

In 1962 or 1966 nearly 17,000 alumni replied to a questionnaire concerning their personal characteristics, their exercise habits, and physician-diagnosed diseases, including coronary heart disease. To assess their adult exercise habits, alumni were asked how many flights of stairs (using ten steps as a flight) they climbed each day, how many city blocks they walked each day, and what sports they played in hours per week. Sports or leisure-time activities were classified as "light" — generally considered to require comparatively little energy output, or about five Kcal per minute (e.g., bowling, baseball, boating, golf, and yardwork) — and as "vigorous" — requiring more energy or about ten Kcal per minute (e.g., running, mountaineering, cross-country skiing, swimming, basketball, and tennis). A physical activity index was devised to provide an estimate of total energy expenditure expressed in kilocalories per week, from stairs climbed, blocks walked, leisure work, and sports played. The physical activity index was divided at 2,000 Kcal per week; alumni whose total energy expenditure was on the low side of this index (fewer than 2,000 Kcal per week) were classified in the low-energy category, and alumni who expended 2,000 or more Kcal per week were placed in the high-energy category. In 1972, a second questionnaire was mailed to each alumnus of classes that entered Harvard from 1916 to 1950 to query men about physician-diagnosed diseases, including coronary heart disease.[229]

Although the range of energy output for the college men was lower than for the longshoremen, findings ran parallel in that the greater the level of energy expended, the lower the risk of heart attack. Alumni who reported expending more than 2,000 Kcal per week had a fifty percent lower risk of heart attack than did their less energetic classmates.

Paffenbarger raised the question whether the differences between the exercising and non-exercising groups are due to "protection or selection." He asked: Is the higher energy output of subjects who exercise hard responsible for lower rates of fatal heart attacks because they are endowed with a "stronger cardio-vascular system" and gravitate toward more active work through life? And do subjects who do not exercise hard have inherently "weaker cardio-vascular systems" and therefore move into less active behavior patterns?

I consider two comments appropriate. First, the terms "strong" and "weak" cardio-vascular systems are meaningless in the context under reference. Subjects who die from myocardial infarction do not die because their cardio-vascular system is "weak." They die because they had been afflicted with a pathological process. This process cannot be reversed through exercise. Secondly, consideration must be given to the fact that physical training enhances performance fitness irrespective of the presence of pathological processes — provided, of course, these processes do not interfere with the body's adaptive responses to exercise. During the early stages of the natural history of the ischemic heart diseases they rarely interfere. One of the most important observations made in our survey of unexpected death during exercise is that fatal seizures revealed at autopsy to have been the result of advanced cardiac disease may occur during strenuous athletic activity — wrestling, swimming, tennis, running, cycling. The cardiac illness did not render impossible attainment and maintenance of a high level of physical performance.

The differences in rates of morbidity and mortality between the exercising and non-exercising groups which Paffenbarger's researches have revealed may well be due to selection and training, not due to a primary "protective" effect of exercise.

This conclusion in no way detracts from the value of exercise in cardiology. The enhancement of performance capacity and the psychological effects of exercise are therapeutic benefits of the utmost importance. No modality of treatment is capable of substituting for them.

The 1952 Olympic Games Survey

At the Olympic Games at Helsinki in 1952 data obtained from all 4,925 participants were evaluated in an attempt to assess the influence upon physical performance capacity of five extraneous determinants: per capita income, death rates, infantile mortality, caloric consumption, and climatic environment.[6]

While Paffenbarger's computations aimed at the identification of a common energy-output-dependent criterium, namely time of onset of fatal heart attacks, the Helsinki Olympic survey was designed to define the role played by extra-somatic modifiers of high energy output capacity, with individually assessed Olympic performances as indicators.

The statistical procedure applied to the grading of every individual performance was based on the assumption that the winner in each Olympic contest had to be allocated 100 points; it being taken for granted that every Olympic Gold Medalist is the world's best performer in his event at the time of his victory, the competitor ranking last was rated 0. It was thus possible to identify on a unified scale performances in different athletic disciplines.

When death rates were computed in juxtaposition to athletic achievement it became apparent that countries with the lowest death rates did best at the Games, while countries with the highest death rates ranked lowest. The predominant causes of death in people under 30 years of age are the infectious diseases from which most people in the poor countries die. Infant mortality is statistically related to athletic achievement. Countries with the highest rates of infant mortality are the ones with the lowest rates of athletic success, and vice versa.

A striking correlation appeared when athletic participation and achievement of nations were evaluated against caloric consumption. Nations which have little to eat are poorly represented among Olympic contestants. They are not likely to produce many winners.

Finally, an attempt was made to ascertain whether athletic performances are modified by climate. The majority of athletes who were successful at the Olympic Games came from the cold zones; the warm and hot zones send only one-sixth of the total number of participants, few among them making the finals.

Julius Cohnheim and William Henry Welch

The issue touched upon in the foregoing pages is of profound theoretical importance. It was first raised more than a century ago by the great pathologist, Julius Cohnheim. His views exerted a lasting influence upon medicine.

Cohnheim held that physiological adaptations are ubiquitously appropriate in that they improve the organism's ability to deal with situations that elicit them; contrariwise, he wrote, the body's responses to pathological processes are arbitrary, often inappropriate, not designed to defend it against disease. He questioned the validity of the time-honored belief that "nature is in possession of unfailing healing powers," and that the physician's task is to strengthen the methods which nature uses to counteract disease processes. This belief, Cohnheim wrote, is fallacious. Teleologically speaking, physiological adjustments "serve their purpose;" while adjustments to pathological processes are "unreliable" — they may be useful, or irrelevant, or deleterious.[18]

At the height of his career, William Henry Welch (1850-1934), the Dean of American Medicine as Simon and James Flexner[230] called him, reviewed the time he spent in Breslau with Cohnheim. He did so twenty years after his return from Germany, when in 1897 he addressed the American Congress of Physicians and Surgeons in Philadelphia. Welch detailed a number of arguments which had convinced Cohnheim that "nature is neither kind nor cruel but simply obedient to law and therefore consistent."

Physiological reactions of the kind Cohnheim had in mind are exemplified by the increase of muscle power in response to demands upon the body's strength, by the improvement of the cardiorespiratory system's capacity to transport oxygen in response to demands upon the body's powers of endurance, or by the progressive differentiation of motor control in response to demands upon manual skill. Contrariwise, the body's adjustments to disease processes do not reveal a like appropriateness: arterial hypertension engenders hypertrophy of the heart muscle of a kind that results in necroses of the enlarged myocardial fibers; the radius of diffusion of oxygen from accompanying capillaries no longer reaches the innermost portions of the pathologically enlarged heart muscle cells. By contrast muscular hypertrophy of the kind that takes place as physiological adjustment, e.g., to a sustained exercise regime, enhances the individual's ability to deal with the situations that gave rise to it. This statement is valid in respect of physiological responses of skeletal as well as myocardial muscle, also in respect of the hypertrophied uterus in pregnancy. Correspondingly opposite examples of "inappropriate" responses are hypertrophic and hyperplastic formation of neoplasms involving muscle tissue, e.g., in uterine myoma.

It is often the body's response to disease processes rather than the disease processes themselves that initiate catastrophies. Cohnheim referred to inflammation as a supposed means of combating infections. Since antiquity physicians have considered inflammation part of the body's effort to ward off the deleterious effects of infectious diseases. Welch described Cohnheim's argument on the issue as follows:

> The more severe and extensive the inflammatory affection, the more serious, as a rule, is the condition of the patient. The surgeon sees his wounds do well or ill according to the character and extent of inflammatory complications. Measures directed to the removal of inflammatory exudation, such as the evacuation of pus from an abscess or an empyema, are the most successful methods of treatment, and the rules are embodied in ancient surgical maxims. How can one conceive of any purpose useful to the patient served by filling the aircells of his lungs with pus-cells, fibrin and red corpuscles in pneumonia, or bathing the brain and spinal cord in serum and pus in meningitis? The closure of pathological defects by new growth of tissue is a process which must be regarded as adaptive. But one would hardly describe as advantageous the scar in the brain which causes epilepsy. If nature has no better weapons than those to fight pneumococcus or meningococcus, it may be asked, what is their use but to drive the devil out with Beelzebub? (S. Flexner, W. James[230])

The term "ischemic heart disease," unknown during Cohnheim's lifetime, pertains to the sequelae of the critical disproportion between demand for and supply of oxygen to the heart muscle. This dispro-portion may threaten the patient's life. It would be quite thinkable for the myocardium to adapt itself to the hypoxic state by utilizing anaerobically produced energy — malignant tumor cells do so. But the myocardial fiber is unable to do likewise. Its reaction to depri-vation of oxygen often results in arrhythmias causing "self-electrocution" of the heart, to use a term applied by the late Claude Beck.[96]

Adaptation in Physiology and Pathology

Cohnheim did not assert that adaptations in pathological pro-cesses are invariably deleterious. We can, he wrote, recognize in the results of morbid processes manifold evidences of adjustment: some are admirably complete; others are adequate but not perfect; but many are associated with such disorder that the element of adapta-tion is conspicuous by its absence. The body simply does not possess weapons designed to defend itself against diseases. The body's weapons are designed to meet physiological demands. What about the role of exercise in cardiac rehabilitation? An attack of myocar-dial infarction may be so severe as to cause the patient's instanta-neous death. Or it may leave him permanently incapacitated. Only if the heart retains sufficient functional reserve to respond to the de-mands of exercise will the patient benefit from a regime of rehabili-tative training. Reference has been made earlier to Kavanagh's studies with "cardiac marathoners" who two years after an attack of myocardial infarction performed on a level of endurance unattain-able to the majority of untrained healthy subjects.[218]

The corresponding opposite to the use of exercise in cardiology is the "abuse of bed rest." Fractures of the neck of the femur occur with conspicuous frequencies in old women, an observation explained in part by their lifestyle which is commonly characterized by physical inactivity. Saltin, Blomquist, Mitchell, et al.[32] demonstrated a sharp decline of cardiovascular efficiency within a few days of bed rest in well trained endurance athletes. "Nature is neither kind nor cruel but simply obedient to law and therefore consistent."

Cohnheim's analysis touches upon traditional beliefs in "the wis-dom of the body."

Paul Ehrlich [17,231]

Paul Ehrlich became acquainted with Cohnheim's ideas which occupied his mind for the rest of his life. Up to 1908, the year he received the Nobel Prize, Ehrlich had pursued his plan to discover specific substances capable of combating pathogenic micro-organisms, the *therapia sterilisans magna* of which he had dreamed since his youth, by adjusting, manipulating, and improving physiologically active substances. When von Behring discovered the diphtheria-antitoxin, it was Ehrlich who noted the substance's therapeutic potency is limited in concentrations in which nature produces it. He set about to make antitoxin available in much higher titers, using new experimental techniques. There is scarcely a normal immunological phenomenon whose therapeutic potentialities Ehrlich had not tried to utilize; but it was only during the last years of his life that he came to rely on non-natural, non-physiological substances, on aniline dyes, on metals and on synthetic chemicals that he succeeded in producing his "magic bullets." The direct line of reagents, of which Sir Henry Dale wrote in recalling his apprenticeship in Ehrlich's institute, "and on the oxygen needs of tissues, through salvarsan to sulphonamides, the antibiotics, and the great modern wealth of directly curative remedies;" this line represents the ultimate application of Cohnheim's thoughts.

Consideration of the role of exercise in cardiology encompasses the role of physiological adaptations in pathological processes. However, the body possesses no weapons of ubiquitous therapeutic effectiveness against diseases. Physiological adaptations often are of advantage to the diseased organism in that they enhance its efficiency, a fact of decisive relevance in all fields of rehabilitation.

The Pritikin Diet

N. Pritikin claims unprecedented therapeutic results through a special diet, more especially with patients with advanced ischemic heart disease.[232] The author's diet guideline is as follows:

Less than 10% fat, 10% to 15% protein, 75% to 80% mainly complex carbohydrates, less than 25 mg of cholesterol (Regression diet), and less than 100 mg of cholesterol (Maintenance diet).

One of Pritikin's patients was a 46-year-old man with severe

peripheral vascular disease "caused by 100% occlusion of both femoral arteries" who could only walk 100 yards but "after two years
on my diet ran a 26 mile marathon." The "100% occlusion of both femoral arteries" is not documented, neither prior to nor at the end of
the two year dietary regimen. The statement that "angiograms after
the marathon were impressive" certainly requires elucidation.

The following quotations are from the same article by Pritikin:

> World class athletes have been on my Regression diet for years,
> two of them for six years each: Robert de Castella, the No. 1
> marathon runner in the world (who beat Alberto Salazar, the No.
> 1 U.S. runner, in April 1983); and David Scott, the No. 1 Iron-
> man Triathlete . . . These examples indicate that both patients
> and physically fit persons can voluntarily comply with my diet
> standards — no institutional environment is needed.
>
> Number 1 marathoner Robert de Castella's father, Rolet . . . was
> medically treated for hypertension, and had a stroke at the age of
> 52 years while running. Nine months later, a myocardial infarc-
> tion incapacitated him for a year with severe angina. Maximum
> medication did not relieve his angina. He then started my Re-
> gression diet. In a short time his angina was gone, and all medi-
> cation was gradually withdrawn. Within two years he ran his first
> marathon. Today at age 59 years, he has run 18 marathons, with
> his best time at three hours. He has been on the Regression diet
> for seven years. (Pritikin[232])

Pritikin's diet is thus claimed to be of major value for endurance
athletes as well as for patients recovering from stroke, myocardial infarction, and angina pectoris.

No diet is able to engender the ability to run 26 miles. The only
way to learn to run for three hours or longer is to train for such a
performance over an extended period. In 1974 Kavanagh, et al.[218]
reported on a group of patients who after recovery from myocardial
infarction had been trained for the marathon. They had not been on
the Pritikin diet.

Claims to the effect that diet can engender the ability to run over
long distances make no sense.

Another important issue at stake is whether pathological processes such as those to which reference is made in the article under
review can be caused to regress or disappear through diet. The chief

claim of a therapeutic effectiveness of Pritikin's diet rests upon an enhancement of physical efficiency. Since all his subjects must have undergone intensive physical training before they could run the marathon or performed well in other physical tasks, one would have expected him to distinguish between the effectiveness of exercise and diet. That exercise improves physical efficiency has been known for a long time. It can safely be assumed that the high physical efficiency of Robert de Castella, Alberto Salazar, David Scott as well as the improved performance capacity of Pritikin's patients was due to exercise.

REFERENCES

1. Buytendijk FJJ, Snapper I: *Ergebnisse sportärztlichen Untersuchungen bei den IX. Olympischen Spielen in Amsterdam 1928.* Berlin, Springer, 1929.
2. Reindell H, Klepzig H, Musshoff K: *"Das Sportherz"* in Bergmann G, Frey GW, Schwiegk H (eds): *Physiologische und pathophysiologische Grundlagen der Grössen — und Formänderungen des Herzens.*
   — *"Das Sportherz"* in Bergmann G, Frey GW, Schwiegk H (eds): *Handbuch der Inneren Medizin,* Vol 9. Berlin, Springer, 1960.
   — and in Reindell H and Roskamm H: *Herzkrankheiten,* Berlin, Springer, 1977 (2nd ed 1983).
3. Abrahams A: "Exercise and cardiac hypertrophy." *The Lancet* ii:565-566, 1946.
4. Abrahams A: "Physical exercise; its clinical implications." *The Lancet* 1133-1137, 1951.
5. Abrahams A: "Physical exercise . . ." *The Lancet* 1187-1192, 1951.
6. Jokl E, Karvonen MJ, Kihlberg J, Koskela A, Noro L: *Sports in the cultural pattern of the world: A Study of the Olympic Games of 1952 at Helsinki.* Institute of Occupational Health (Monograph), Helsinki, Finland, 1956, pp 1-116.
7. Moritz AR, Zamcheck N: "Sudden and unexpected deaths of young soldiers." *Arch Path* 42:459-494, 1946.
8. Jokl E, McClellan JT: "Exercise and cardiac death." *Medicine and Sport,* Vol 5. Basel, Karger, 1971.
9. White PD, Pomeroy WC: "Bradycardia below rates of 40 in athletes, especially in long distance runners." *JAMA* 120(8):642, 1942.
10. White PD, Gertler MM: *Athletic Activity and Occupation in Coronary Heart Disease in Young Adults.* Harvard University Press, 1954.
11. White PD: "Preface" in Brunner D, Jokl E (eds): *Physical Activity and Aging.* Basel, Karger, 1970.
12. Currens JH, White PD: "Half a century of running; clinical, physiologic and autopsy findings in the case of Clarence DeMar ('Mr. Marathon')." *N Engl J Med* 265:988-993, 1961.
13. Jokl E: "Syncope in athletes." *Manpower,* South African Government Publication, Vol 5-6. (1-2): 1-198, 1947.
14. Rokitansky C: *A Manual of Pathological Anatomy,* Vol 1-4. London, The Sydenham Society, 1849-1985.

14. Rokitansky C: *A Manual of Pathological Anatomy,* Vol 1-4. London, The Sydenham Society, 1849-1985.
15. Editorial: *The Lancet* 1258, 1938.
16. Jokl E: "Effect of sports and athletics on the cardiovascular system." *Cardiology.* Encyclopedia of the Cardiovascular System. American College of Cardiology, 1961.
17. Jokl E: "Paul Ehrlich — Scientist." *Bulletin of N. Y. Academy of Medicine,* 30:12, Dec 1954.
18. Cohnheim J: *Vorlesungen über allgemeine Pathologie, in Handbuch für Arzte and Studierende.* Berlin, Verlag von August Hirschwald, 1877.
19. Friend GE: "Exercise and Heart Strain." *Practitioner* 135:265-271, Sept 1935.
20. Henschen SE: *Eine medizinische Sportstudie; Skidlauf und Skidwettlauf, Mitteilungen aus der Medizinischen Klinik zu Upsala, Schweden,* Vol II, 1899.
21. Keul J, Dickhuth HH, Lehmann M, et al: "The Athlete's Heart — Haemodynamics and structure." *Int J Sports Med* 3:33-43, 1982.
22. Davies KJA, Packer L, Brooks GA: "Biochemical Adaptation of mitochondria, muscle, and whole-animal respiration to endurance training." *Arch Biochem Biophys* 209(2);539-554, 1981.
23. Rost W, Hollmann W: "Athlete's Heart." *Int J Sports Med* 4(3):147-200, 1983.
24. Schamroth L, Jokl E: "Marked sinus and A-V nodal bradycardia with interference-dissociation in an athlete." *J Sports Med Phys Fitness* 9(2):128-129, 1969.
25. Raab W: *Prevention of Ischemic Heart Disease.* Springfield, Charles C Thomas, 1964.
26. Morganroth J, Maron BJ, Henry WL, et al: "Comparative left ventricular dimensions in trained athletes." *Ann Intern Med* 82:521-524, 1975.
27. Morganroth J, Maron BJ: "The athlete's heart syndrome: a new perspective." *Ann NY Acad Sci* 301:931-941, 1977.
28. Maron BJ, Roberts WC, Edwards JE, et al: "Sudden in patients with hypertrophic cardiomyopathy: characterization of 26 patients without functional limitation." *Am J Cardiol* 41(5):803-810, 1978.
29. Maron BJ, Roberts WC, McAllister HA, et al: "Sudden death in young athletes." *Circulation* 62(2):218-229, 1980.
30. Linzbach AJ: *"Die pathologische Anatomie der Herzinsuffizienz"* in Bergmann G, Frey GW, Schwiegk H (eds): *Handbuch der Inneren Medizin,* Vol 9. Berlin, Springer, 1960.
31. Astrand PO, Engstrom L, Eriksson BO, et al: "Girl Swimmers." *Acta Paediatr Scand* (Suppl) 147:1-75, 1963.
32. Saltin B, Blomquist G, Mitchell JH, et al: *Response to Exercise After Bed Rest and After Training: A Longitudinal Study of Adaptive Changes in Oxygen Transport and Body Composition.* American Heart Association Monograph, No 23. New York, 1968.
33. Pyorala K, Karvonen MJ, Taskinen P, et al: "Cardiovascular studies on former endurance athletes" in Karvonen MJ, Barry AJ (eds): *Physical Activity and the Heart.* Springfield, Charles C Thomas, 1967, 301-309.

34. Pyorala K, Karvonen MJ, Taskinen P, et al: "Cardiovascular studies on former endurance athletes." *Am J Cardiol* 20(2):191-205, 1967.
35. Karvonen MJ, Klemola H, Virkajarvi J, et al: "Longevity of endurance skiers." *Med Sci Sports* 6:49-51, 1974.
36. Rook AF: "Flying, medical aspects" in *Medical Annual*, London, 1940.
37. Jokl E, McClellan JT: "Exercise and Cardiac Death." *JAMA* 213:1489-1491, August 31, 1970.
38. Roskamm H, Gohlke H, et al: *Int J Sports Med* 5:1-10, 1984.
39. Jokl E, Newman B: "Death of a Wrestler" in Jokl E, McClellan JT (eds): *Exercise and Cardiac Death*, Vol 5: *Medicine and Sport*. Basel, Karger, 1971: 81-90.
40. Jokl E, Greenstein J: "Fatal coronary sclerosis in a boy of ten years." *The Lancet* 147:659, 1944.
41. Jokl E, McClellan JT: "Sudden Cardiac Death of Pilots in Flight" in Jokl E, McClellan JT (eds): *Exercise and Cardiac Death*, Vol 5: *Medicine and Sport*. Basel, Karger, 1971: 115-165.
42. Tunstall-Pedoe D: "Exercise and Sudden Death." *Brit J Sports Med* 12:215-219, 1979.
43. Waller BF, Roberts WC: "Sudden death while running in conditioned runners aged 40 years or over." *Am J Cardiol* 45:1292-1297, 1979.
44. Rayman RB, McNaughton GB: "Sudden incapacitation: ISAF experience 1970-80." *Aviat, Sp and Environ Med* 161-164, 1983.
45. Giknis FL, Holt DE, Whiteman HW, et al: Myocardial infarction in twenty-year-old identical twins" in Jokl E, McClellan JT (eds): *Exercise and Cardiac Death*, Vol 5: *Medicine and Sport*. Basel, Karger, 1971:159-165.
46. Jokl E: "Twin Research in Cardiology with a Comment on the Role of Genetic Design in Physiology and Pathology." *Twin Research: Clinical Studies*. 49-55. Alan R. Liss, New York, 1978.
47. Handler JB, Asay RW, Warren SE, et al: "Symptomatic coronary artery disease in a marathon runner." *JAMA* 248(6):717-719, 1982.
48. Jokl E: "Sudden Death after Exercise Due to Myocarditis" in Jokl E, McClellan JT (eds): *Exercise and Cardiac Death*, Vol 5: *Medicine and Sport*. Basel, Karger, 1971: 115-165.
49. Kolb G: *"Gonorrhoische Endokarditis bei Meistern im Wettrudern"* in *Beitrage zur Physiologie maximaler Muselarbeit*. Berlin, S Braun, 1898:103F.
50. Hanson PG, Vander Ark CR, Besozzi MC, et al: "Myocardial infarction in a national class swimmer." *JAMA* 248(18):2313-2314, 1982.
51. Kimbiris D, Segal BL, Munir M, et al: "Myocardial infarction in patients with normal patent coronary arteries as visualized by cinarteriography." *Am J Cardiol* 29:290-291, 1972.
52. Green LH, Cohen SI, Kurland G: Fatal myocardial infarction in marathon racing." *Ann Intern Med* 84:705-706, 1976.
53. Connor RCR: "Sudden death after exertion in apparently healthy boy." *Br Med J* 1:30-31, 1969.
54. Karjalainen J, Heikkila J: "Myocardial infarction or acute myopericarditis (letter)." *JAMA* 249(22):3018, 1983.

55. Jokl E, Parade GW: *"Zur Frage der Beurteilung von Herzfällen in der sportärztlichen Praxis." Med Klin* 29:1070-1074, 1933.
56. Jokl E, Suzman MM: "Aortic regurgitation and mitral stenosis in a marathon runner." *JAMA* 114:467-470, 1940.
57. Warfield LM: "The heart and athletics: modern concepts of cardiovascular disease." Monthly Publication of Am Heart Assoc 3(5), 1934.
58. Lynch P: "Soldiers, Sport, and Sudden Death." *The Lancet* 1235-1237, June 7, 1980.
59. Jokl E: "Exercise and cardiac death" in *Proceedings, International Conference on Sports Cardiology.* Rome, Aulo Gagi, 1980.
60. Rost W, Hollmann W: "Athlete's heart." *Int J Sports Med* 4(3):147-200, 1983.
61. Jokl E, MacIntosh RH: "Sudden death of young athlete from rupture of ascending aorta." *The Lancet* i:54-55, 1950.
62. Bonnet LM: *"Sur la lesion diet stenose congenitale de l'aorte dans le region de l'isthme." Rev de Med Pat* XXIII:108,255,335,418,481, 1903.
63. Hart C: *"Uber die totale Obliteration des Aortenisthmus." Med Klin* 16:1337, 1920.
64. Wasastjerna E: *"Ein Fall von Aortenruptur nach Schlittschuhlaufen bei einem scheinbar gesunden 13 jährigen Knaben." Ztschr f Klin Med* 49:405-410, 1903.
65. Jores L: *"Arterien"* in Henke F, Lubarsch O (eds): *Handbuch der speziellen pathologischen Anatomie und Histologie,* Vol II, Berlin, Springer, 1924: 608-786.
66. Henke F, Lubarsch O (eds): *Handbuch der speziellen pathologischen Anatomie und Histologie,* Vol II, Berlin, Springer, 1924.
67. Taussig H: *Congenital Malformations of the Heart.* Cambridge, Harvard Univ Press, 1947.
68. Keith A: "Malformation of the heart." *The Lancet* i:14-21, 1909.
69. Mönckeberg JG: *"Die Missbildungen des Herzens"* in Henke F, Lubarsch O (eds): *Handbuch der speziellen pathologischen Anatomie und Histologie,* Vol II, Berlin, 1934.
70. Craven D, Jokl E: "Medical research in physical education: case histories." *South African Med J* 19:246-248, 1945.
71. Jokl E, Cluver EH: "Sudden death of a rugby international after a test game" in Jokl E, McClellan JT (eds): *Exercise and Cardiac Death,* Basel, Karger, 1971:153-158.
72. Editorial: "Aortic Hypoplasia: a cause of death?" *The Lancet* 408, 1969.
73. Paltauf A: *"Ueber die Beziehung der Thymus zum plötzlichen Tod." Wien Klin Wchnschr* 2(46):877-881, 1889.
74. Paltauf A: *Ueber die Beziehung der Thymus zum plotzlichen Tod." Wien Klin Wchnschr* 3(9):172-175, 1890.
75. Carr JL: "Status thymico-lymphaticus." *The Journal of Pediatrics* 27(1):1-43, 1945.
76. Jokl E, McClellan JT, Williams WC, Gouze FJ and Bartholomew RD: "Congenital Anomaly of Left Coronary Artery in Young Athletes." *Cardiologia* 49:253-258, 1966.
77. Jokl E, McClellan JT and Ross GD: "Congenital Anomaly of Left Coronary Artery in Young Athlete." *JAMA* 182:572-573, November 3, 1962.

78. McClellan JT, Jokl E: "Congenital anomalies of coronary arteries as cause of sudden death associated with physical exertion." *Amer J Clin Pathol* 50(2):229-233, 1968.

79. Virmani R, Chun PKC, Goldstein RE, et al: "Acute takeoffs of the coronary arteries along the aortic wall and congenital coronary ostial valve-like ridges: Association with sudden death." *J Am College Cardiol* 3(3):766-771, 1984.

80. Wolf PL, Bing R: "The smallest tumor which causes sudden death." *JAMA* 194:674-675, 1965.

81. Jokl E, McClellan JT: "Exercise and cardiac death." *JAMA* 213(9):1489-1491, 1970.

82. Case Record, Weekly Clinicopathological Exercises. *N Engl J Med* 308:206-214, 1983.

83. James TN: "Primary and Secondary Cardioneuropathies and their Functional Significance." *Journal of the American College of Cardiology* Nov 1983: 983-1002.

84. James TN, Friggatt P, Marshall TK: "Sudden death in young athletes." *Ann Int Med* 67(5):1013-1021, 1967.

85. James TN, Pearce WN, Givhan EG Jr: "Sudden death while driving." *Am J Cardiol* 45:1095-1102, 1980.

86. Bharati S, Bauernfeind R, Miller LB, et al: "Sudden death in three teenagers: conduction system studies." *J Amer Coll Cardiol* 1(3):879-886, 1983.

87. Green JR, Krovetz LJ, Shanklin DR, et al: "Sudden unexpected death in three generations" in Jokl E, McClellan JT (eds): *Exercise and Cardiac Death,* Vol 5: *Medicine and Sport.* Basel, Karger, 1971: 166-175.

88. Baim DD, Harrison DC: "Nonatherosclerotic coronary heart disease (including coronary artery spasm)" in Hurst JW (ed): *The Heart.* McGraw-Hill (5th ed), 1982.

89. Moritz AR: "Injuries of the heart and pericardium by physical violence" in Gould SE (ed): *Pathology of the Heart and Blood Vessels.* Springfield, Charles C Thomas, 1968.

90. Jokl E: *"Tod beim Sport"* in *Funktionelle Krankheitsbilder beim Sport.* Schweiz, Medizin Wschr 63:49,1278-1282, 1933.

91. Weber EF: *"Uber ein Verfahren, den Kreislauf des Blutes u. die Function des Herzens willkürlich zu unterbrechen: Ber u. d. Verhand. d." Sächs Gesel d Wissenschaft* zu Leipzig, 1850, 29.

92. Schlomka G: *"Commotio Cordis und ihre Folgen (Die) Einwirkung stumpfer Brustwandtraumen auf das Herz)"* Ergebn d inn Med, u Kinderh 47:1-91, 1934.

93. Deutsch F: *"Sekundenherztod im Boxkampf durch Commotio cordis (Ein Beitrag zur Frage des Sportherzens)."* Wien Arch f Inn Med 20:279-286, 1930.

94. Jankovitch L: *"Suites mortelles d'un combat de boxe."* Ann de med leg 15:795-799, 1935.

95. Warburg E: *Subacute and Chronic Pericardial and Myocardial Lesions Due to Nonpenetrating Traumatic Injuries.* Copenhagen and London, 1938.

96. Beck CS: "Contusions of heart." *JAMA* 104:109-114, 1935.

 97. Moullin F: Quoted from "Traumatic injury of heart." *Clin Soc* London. *The Lancet* i:314, 1897.
 98. Schorre E: *"Über Herzrupturen nach Bauchtraumen." Ztschr f Kreislaufforsch* 27:577-583, 1935.
 99. Schlomka G: *"Experimentelle Untersuchungen über den Einfluss stumpfer Brustkorbtraumen auf das Herz; der chronische postkommotionelle Herzschaden." Ztschr f d ges exper Med* 93:751-774, 1934.
100. Schlomka G: *"Experimentelle Untersuchungen über den Einfluss stumpfer Brustkorbtraumen auf das Herz; das besondere Verhalten sensibilisierter Tiere." Ztschr f d ges exper Med* 92:552-572, 1934.
101. Schlomka G, Schmitz M: *"Experimentelle Untersuchungen über den Einfluss stumpfer Brustkorbtraumen auf das Herz: die acute traumatische Herzdilatation." Ztschr f d ges exper Med* 90:301-318, 1933.
102. Jokl E, Melzer L: "Acute fatal non-traumatic collapse during work and sport." *South African J Med Sc* 5:4-14, 1940.
103. Parsons-Smith G, Williams D: "Cerebral embolism following contusion of the heart." *Br Med J* 1:10-12, 1949.
104. Boyd AM, Jepson RP: "External iliac artery thrombosis." *Br Med J* 1:1457-1460, 1950.
105. Glancy DL, Yarnell PH, Roberts WC: "Traumatic left ventricular aneurysm" in Jokl E, McClellan JT (eds): *Exercise and Cardiac Death.* Basel, Karger, 1971.
106. Weiss S: "Instantaneous 'physiological' death." *New Engl J Med* 223(20):293-297, 14 Nov 1940.
107. Jokl E: *The Clinical Physiology of Physical Fitness and Rehabilitation.* Springfield, Charles C Thomas, 1958.
108. Bernard C: *an Introduction to the Study of Experimental Medicine.* New York, Macmillan Co, 1927.
109. Abrahams A: "Athletics." *Brit Encycl Med Prac,* London, 1950.
110. Wyndham CH: "Heatstroke and hypothermia in marathon runners" in Milvey P (ed): *The Marathon: Physiological, Medical, Epidemiological, and Psychological Studies.* Ann Ny Acad Sci, 1977: 128-138.
111. Sohar E, Michaeli D, Waks U, et al: "Heatstroke caused by dehydration and physical effort." *Arch Intern Med* 122:159-169, 1968.
112. Shibolet S, Lancaster MO, Danon Y: "Heat stroke: a review." *Aviat Sp Environ Med* 280-301, 1976.
113. Schrier RW, Henderson HS, Tisher CC, et al: "Nephropathy associated with heat stress and exercise (XIII)" in Jokl E, McClellan JT (eds): *Exercise and Cardiac Death,* Vol 5: *Medicine and Sport.* Basel, Karger, 1971: 121-147.
114. Parsons KT, Anderson RJ: "Pathogenesis and Management of Renal Failure due to Physical Exertion and Exertional Heatstroke" in *Internal Medicine for the Specialist,* Vol 5. June 7 1984.
115. Graber CD, Reinhold RB, Breman JG, et al: "Fatal heat stroke: circulating endotoxin and gram-negative sepsis as complications." *JAMA* 216(7): 1195-1196, 1971.

116. Pugh LG: "Accidental hypothermia in walkers, climbers and campers: report to the Medical Commission on Accident Prevention." *Brit Med J* 1(5480):123-129, 1966.

117. Pugh LG, Edholm OG, Rox RH, et al: "A physiological study of channel swimming." *Clin Sci* 19:257-273, 1960.

118. Gauer OH, Thron HL: "Postural changes in the circulation." *Handbook of Physiology Circul* (III), 1965.

119. Humboldt, A von: *"Die Besteigung des Chimborazo"* in Douglas Botting's biography. Prestel, Munich, 1973: 173-194.

120. Mosso A: *Der Mensch auf den Hochalpen*. Leipzig, Velt & Co, 1899.

121. Bert P: "Barometric Pressure." *Researches in Experimental Physiology.* Translated from the French by MA and FA Hitchcock. Columbus, Ohio, 1943.

122. Henderson Y: *Adventures in Respiration*. London, Bailliere, Tindall & Cox, 1938.

123. Lewis T: *The soldier's heart and the effort syndrome*. London, His Majesty's Stationery Office, 1918.

124. Jokl E: "Medical Problems of Aviation." *J Roy Army Med Corps.* London, John Bale Sons & Curnow, Ltd, 1939.

125. Bürger M, Bürger H, Petersen PF: *"Die Pressdruckprobe als Herzleistungsprüfung."* *Arbeitsphysiol* 1:614-624, 1929.

126. Rook AF: "Flying, Medical Aspects" in *Medical Annual*, London, 1940.

127. Deutsch F: *"Die Herzgrössenschwankungen, speziell die deminutio cordis, unmittelbar nach sportlichen Leistungen"* in Buytendijk FJJ (ed): *Ergebnisse der Sportärztlichen Untersuchungen bei den IX. Olympischen Spielen.* Berlin, Verlag von Julius Springer, 1929: 82-99.

128. Gauer OH: *"Kreislauf des Blutes"* in Gauer OH (ed): *Physiologie des Menschen, Bd 3: Herz und Kreislauf,* Munich, Urban & Schwarzenberg, 1972.

129. Jokl P, Jokl E: "Running and swimming world records." *Brit J Sports Med* 10(4):1976 (Dec) Festschrift for 90th birthday of Professor A.V. Hill.

130. Eichna LW, Horvath SM, Bean WB: "Post-exertional orthostatic hypotension." *Am J Med Sc* 213:614-654, 1947.

131. Schlesinger A: "Life-threatening 'Vagal Reaction' to physical fitness tests." *JAMA* 226(9):1119, 1973.

132. Biggs R: *Human Blood Coagulation Haemostasis and Thrombosis*, (2nd ed), Oxford Blackwell Scientific Pub, 1976.

133. Lennox WG, Gibbs FA, Gibbs EL: "Relationship of unconsciousness to cerebral blood flow and to anoxaemia." *Arch Neurol and Psychiat* 34:1001-1013, 1935.

134. Weber EF: *"Über ein Verfahren, den Kreislauf des Blutes und die Funktion des Herzens willkürlich zu unterbrechen."* *Berichte über die Verhandlungen der Königlich Sächsischen Gessellschaft der Wissenschaften, zu* Leipzig, 1850: 20.

135. Visscher MB: "Restriction of coronary flow as general factor in heart failure." *JAMA* 113:987-990, 1939.

136. Comptom DP, Hill McN, Sinclair JD: "Weight-lifters' blackout." *The Lancet* i:1234-1237, 1973.

108   *Sudden Death of Athletes*

Bibliography follows

137. Bürger M: *"Über die Bedeutung des intrapulmonalen Drucks für den Kreislauf und den Mechanismus des Kollapses bei akuten Anstrengungen."* *Klin Wchnschr* 5:777-780; 825-829, 1926.
138. Craig AB: "Underwater swimming and loss of consciousness." *JAMA* 176(4):255-258, 1961.
139. Jokl E: "Altitude diseases." *New Engl J Med* 280(25):1420-1422, 1969.
140. de Acosta J: *Historia Natural y Moral de las Indias, en que Se Tratan Las Casa Notables del Cielo, y Elementos, Metales, Plantas y Animales de las: Y los ritos, y ceremonias leyes, y govierno, y guerras de los Indios.* Seville, Juan de Leoy, 1590.
141. Kronecker H: *Die Bergkrankheit.* Berlin & Wien, 1903.
142. Zuntz H, Loewy A, Muller F, et al: *Höhenklima and Bergwanderungen.* Deutsches Verlagshaus Bond & Co, 1906.
143. Jokl E, Jokl P: "Indisposition after running" in Jokl E, Jokl P (eds): *International Research on Sport and Physical Education*, Springfield, Thomas, 1964: 692-689.
144. Houston CS: "Acute pulmonary edema of high altitude." *N Engl J Med* 263:964-968, 1960.
145. Dalessio DJ: "Effort migraine." *Headache* 14(1): 53, 1974.
146. Jokl E: *"Die Sportkrankheit."* *Klinische Wochenschrift* 21:984-985, Berlin, 24 Mai 1930.
147. Appenzeller O, et al: *Sports Medicine: Fitness Training, Injuries.* (2nd ed) Urban and Schwarzenberg, Baltimore-Munich, 1983.
148. Loewy A: *Physiologie des Höhenklimas.* Berlin, Julius Springer, 1932.
149. Darling RC: "Heat sickness, high altitude sickness, motion sickness" in Loeb C (ed): *Textbook of Medicine.* Philadelphia, W.B. Saunders, 1963.
150. Forwand AS, Landowne M, Follansbee JN, et al: "Effect of acetazolamide in acute mountain sickness." *N Engl J Med* 279:839-845, 1968.
151. Singh I, Khanna PK, Srivastava MC, et al: "Acute mountain sickness." *N Engl J Med* 280:175-184, 1969.
152. Seelinger DF, Coin GC, Carlow TJ: "Effort headache with cerebral infarction." *Headache* 15(2):142-145, 1975.
153. Miller RG: "Transient focal cerebral ischemia after extreme exercise" *Headache* 17:196-197, 1977.
154. Matthews WB: "Footballer's migraine." *Br Med J* 2:326-327, 1972.
155. Jokl E: *Zuzammenbrüche beim Sport.* Manzsche Verlags und Universitäts-Buchhandlung, Wien, 1936.
156. Wilson SAK: *Neurology.* London, Edward Arnold & Co, Vol II:1545-1560, 1940.
157. Wilder J: *"Narkolepsie"* in Bumke O and Foerster O (eds): *Handbuch der Neurologie* vol XVII, Springer, Berlin, 1935.
158. Jokl E: "8.90: Bob Beamon's World Record Jump." *Olympic Review, I.O.C.,* Lausanne, Nov/Dec, 1972.
159. Magoun HW: *The Waking Brain.* Springfield, Thomas, 1972.
160. Loewy A, Jokl E: *"Abschwächung von Reflexen im Höhenklima."* *Z Neur* 145:733, 1933.

161. Johnson BL, Jokl E, Jokl P: "The effect of exercise upon the duration of the triceps surae stretch reflex." *J Assoc Phys Ment Rehab* 17(6), 1963.

162. Gowers WR: *Epilepsy and Other Chronic Convulsive Diseases: Their Causes, Symptoms and Treatment,* 2. Aufg. London, Churchill, 1901.

163. Phillips J, Horner B, Doorly T, et al: "Cerebrovascular accident in a 14-year-old marathon runner." *BMJ* 286:351-2, 1983.

164. Chester JF, Conlon CP: "Some cerebrovascular complications of exercise." *Brit J Sports Med* 17(4):143-144, 1983.

165. Hermann K, McGregor AR: "Cerebral hemorrhage from rupture of intra-cerebral aneurysm in a child." *Br Med J* 1:523-525, 1940.

166. Kelly WF, Roussak J: "Stroke while jogging." *Brit J Sports Med* 14:229-230, 1980.

167. Muir AL, Percy-Robb IW, Davidson JA, et al: "Physiological aspects of the Edinburgh Commonwealth Games." *The Lancet* 2:1125-1128, 1970.

168. Zinsser H: *Resistance to Infectious Diseases.* New York, MacMillan, 1931.

169. *The Times,* London. 15 Sept 1947.

170. Gore I, Saphir O: "Myocarditis: a classification of 1,402 cases." *Am Heart J* 34:827-830, 1947.

171. Jokl E: "Immunological status of athletes" in *The Role of Exercise in Internal Medicine,* Vol 10: *Medicine and Sport,* Basel, Karger, 1977.

172. Jokl E: *"Serologische Untersuchungen an Sportsleuten." Z Exp Med* 77:65-101, 1931.

173. Green RL, Kaplan SS, Rabin BS, et al: "Immune function in marathon runners." *Ann Allergy* 47(2):73-75, 1981.

174. Jokl E: *"Über Beeinflussung der immunbiologischen Normalstruktur des menschlichen Serums durch Körperarbeit; Das Verhalten der hämolytischen Kraft des aktiven Serums sowie des Normal-Hammelblutamboceptors im aktivierten Serum." Ztschr f d ges Neurol u Psychiat* 129:460-471, 1930.

175. Cannon WB: *Bodily Changes in Pain, Hunger, Fear, and Rage.* New York, D. Appleton & Co, 1915.

176. de Rudder B, Petersen GA: *"Steigert körperliche Anstrengung die Disposition zu epidemischer Kinderlähmung?" Klin Wchnschr.* May 17 1938: 699-702.

177. Levinson SO, Milzer A, Lewin P: "Effect of fatigue, chilling and mechanical trauma in resistance to experimental poliomyelitis." *Am J Hyg* 42:204-213, 1945.

178. Russell WR: "Poliomyelitis, pre-paralytic stage, and the effect of physical activity on the severity of paralysis." *Br Med J* 2:1023-1028, 1947.

179. Hargreaves ER: "Poliomyelitis: effects of exertion during the pre-paralytic stage." *Br Med J* 2:1021-1022, 1948.

180. Russell WR: "Paralytic poliomyelitis — early symptoms and effect of physical activity on course of disease." *Br Med J* 1:465-471, 1949.

181. Williams, ECP: "A second attack of poliomyelitis." *Br med J* 2:1062-1063, 1951.

182. Weinstein L: "Poliomyelitis: a persistent problem." *N Engl J Med* 288:370-372, 1973.

183. Krikler DM, Zilberg B: "Activity and hepatitis." *The Lancet* 2:1046-1047, 1966.

184. Morse LJ: "The Holy Cross College football team hepatitis outbreak." *JAMA* 219:706-708, 1972.

185. Baron RC, Milford HH, Kleeman K, et al: "Aseptic meningitis among members of a high school football team." *JAMA* 248(14):1724-1727, 1962.

186. Evans AS: "Resumption of exercise after infectious mononucleosis." *JAMA* 229(7):847, 1974.

187. Jokl E: "Physical Fitness and Susceptibility to Infections." *J Assoc Phys Ment Rehab* 13:5, Sept/Oct 1959.

188. Dormer BA, Friedlander J, Jokl E: "Physical efficiency and pulmonary tuberculosis." *South African J Sci* XXXVIII:267-277, 1942.

189. Editorial: "Vaccinia after boxing." *The Lancet* i:819, 1948.

190. Ruch DM: "Dermatological disorders in athletes." *Wisc Med J* 63:367-370, 1964.

191. Porter PS, Banghman RD: "Epidemiology of Herpes Simplex among Wrestlers." *JAMA* Nov 29 1965.

192. Wheeler CE, Cabaniss WH: "Epidemic Cutaneous Herpes Simplex in Wrestlers *(herpes Gladiatorium)*." *JAMA* Nov 29 1965.

193. Glezen P, Dewalt J, Lindway R, et al: "Epidemic of pyodermia caused by nephritogenic streptococci in college athletes." *The Lancet* i:301-304, 1972.

194. Sieler H: "*Hautkrankheiten und Sport.*" *Med und Sport* 23(9):285-293, 1983.

195. White WB, et al: "Transmission of Herpes Simplex Virus Type 1 Infection in Rugby Players." *JAMA* 252(4):533-535, July 27 1984.

196. Clarke D, Jokl E, Kloppers PJ: "Physical health and social status of good and bad pupils." *The Journal of Education*, 1946.

197. Milne FT, Cluver EH, Suzman H, Jokl E, et al: "Does a physiological correlation exist between basic intelligence and physical efficiency of school children?" *J Gen Psychol* 63:131-140, 1943.

198. Powell DB: *Equine Vet J* 1:1-4, 1978.

199. Holden C: *Science* 200:14, April 1978.

200. Cerva L, Novak K, Culbertson CG: "An outbreak of acute fatal amebic meningoencephalitis." *Am J Epidem* 88:436-444, 1968.

201. Ruma RJ, Ferrell HW, Nelson EC, et al: "Swimmer's itch." *JAMA* 167:617, 1958.

202. Butt CG: "Primary amebic meningoencephalitis." *N Engl J Med* 274:1473-1476, 1966.

203. *Morbidity and Mortality Weekly Report, U.S. Center for Disease Control*, Dept HEW, Atlanta, Georgia, Sept 15 1978.

204. Rosenberg ML, Hazlet KK, et al: "Shigellosis from Swimming." *JAMA* 236, Oct 18 1976.

205. Parsons MA, Anderson PB, Williams BT: "An 'unavoidable' Death in a People's Marathon." *Brit J Sports Med* 18(1):38-39, March 1984.

206. Dodek A, Demots H, Antonovic J, et al: "Echiuococcus of the heart; an unusual tumor of the heart and liver." *Am J Cardiol* 30:293-297, 1972.

207. Limacher MC, McEntee CW, Attat M, et al: "Cardiac echinoccal cyst: diagnosis by two dimensional echocardiography." *J Amer Coll Cardiol* 2(3):574-577, 1983.

208. Evans RR: "Cysticercosis in a successful athlete." *Trans R Soc Trop Med Hyg* 32:549-550, 1939.
209. Cussen J: *Proc Brit Assoc Sport and Medicine.* St. Mary's Hosp Med School, London, 1957.
210. Hanley DF: "Medical care of the U.S. Olympic team." *JAMA* 236:147-148, 1976.
211. MaeGraith B: *"Unde venis?" The Lancet* i:401-404, 1963.
212. Hornblow PJ: "Mountaineers and medicine." *The Lancet* i:817-819, 1960.
213. Thümmler M: *"Zur Häufigkeitsverteilung von Krankheiten des Atmungssystems bei regalmässig tranierenden Sportlern." Medizin und Sport* 4:114-117, 1983.
214. Linzbach AJ: *"Das Altern des Menschlichen Herzens"* in *Handbuch der Allgemeinen Pathologie* 1:4, Springer, Berlin, 1972.
215. ----------: *"Die Alternsveränderungen des menschlichen Herzens;* I. *Das Herzgewicht im Alter." Klin Wschr* 51, Springer-Verlag, 1973.
216. Jokl E: *Alter und Leistung,* (Monograph, pp 1-75). Springer-Verlag, Berlin-Heidelberg, 1954.
217. Jung K: *Phänomen 100 Km Lauf, Physiologische, Medizinische und Psychologische Aspekte.* München, Schwarzek Verlag, 1981.
218. Kavanagh T, Shepard RJ, Pondit V: "Marathon running after myocardial infarction." *JAMA* 229(12):1602-1605, 1974.
219. Jokl E: "Physical activity and ageing." *Ann Sports Med* 1(2):43-48, 1983.
220. Robinson S: "Experimental studies of physical fitness in relation to age." *Arbeitsphysiologie* 10:251, 1938.
221. Hollmann W: "Performance behavior and trainability in old age" in *IXX International Congress of Gerontology,* Abstracts. Vol 2.
222. Shock N, Strehler BL: "The physiology of aging." *Sci Am* 206:1-100, 1962.
223. Mohler SR: "Reasons for eliminating the 'age 60' regulation for airline pilots." *Aviat Sp Environ Med* 52, 1981.
224. Kohn R: "Cause of death in very old people." *JAMA* 247:2793-2797, 1982.
225. Yudkin J: "Sugar and coronary thrombosis." *Postgrad Med* 44:67-70, Aug 1968.
226. Greenfield JG, Blackwood W, McMenemy WA, et al: *Neuropathology.* London, Edward Arnold, 1961.
227. Keys A: "Physical Activity and the Epidemiology of Coronary Heart Disease" in *Physical Activity and Aging,* Vol 4. *Medicine and Sport.* Karger, Basel/New York, 1970:250-266.
228. Paffenbarger RS, Wing AL, Hyde RT: "Physical activity as an index of heart attack risk in college alumni." *Am J Epidemiol* 108:161-175, 1978.
229. Thomas GS, Lee PR, Franks P, et al: *Exercise and Health: The Evidence and the Implications.* Cambridge, Oelgeschlager, Gunn & Hain, 1981:35.
230. Flexner S, James W: *Henry Welch and the Heroic Age of American Medicine.* New York, Viking Press, 1941.
231. Ehrlich P: *Eine Darstellung seines Wissenschaftlichen Wirkens.* Verlag von Gustav Fischer, 1914.
232. Pritikin N: "Letter to the editor." *JAMA* 251(9): 1160-1161, 1984.

233. Jokl E: *Heart and Sport.* Springfield, IL, Charles C Thomas, 1964.
234. Jokl E: "Olympic Medicine and Sports." *Annals of Sports Med.,* I/4. 1984, 127-169.
235. Jokl E: *The Medical Aspect of Boxing.* Pretoria, JL v Schaik, 1941.
236. Jokl E (Editor): *The Role of Exercise in Internal Medicine,* Basel, Karger, 1974.
237. Jokl E, Ehrlich P: "Man and Scientist." *Bull. N.Y. Acad. Med.,* Dec. 1954, 968-975.

AUTHOR INDEX

SUBJECT INDEX